LILY BENNETT

Hypothyroidism Treatment Revolution

A Comprehensive Guide to Managing Symptoms, Diet, and Thyroid Health

Contents

Introduction

Imagine waking up every day feeling like you haven't slept at all, your body weighed down by an invisible force that saps your energy and dulls your mind. You struggle to focus, your mood swings wildly, and despite eating healthily and exercising, you continue to gain weight. This is the reality for millions of people suffering from hypothyroidism, a condition where the thyroid gland doesn't produce enough thyroid hormones, leading to a myriad of physical and mental health issues.

Hypothyroidism is more than just a medical condition; it's a life-altering challenge that affects every aspect of daily living. The thyroid gland, a small butterfly-shaped organ located at the base of the neck, plays a crucial role in regulating metabolism, energy production, and hormonal balance. When it fails to function correctly, the impact can be profound and far-reaching.

The symptoms of hypothyroidism can vary widely, affecting both physical and mental health. Common physical symptoms include fatigue, weight gain, cold intolerance, dry skin, and hair loss. Mental health symptoms can range from depression and anxiety to cognitive impairments like memory loss and difficulty concentrating. The condition can also lead to complications such as high cholesterol, heart disease, and infertility if left untreated.

Purpose of the Book

"Hypothyroidism Treatment Revolution: A Comprehensive Guide to Managing Symptoms, Diet, and Thyroid Health" is designed to be a beacon of hope and a practical roadmap for those navigating the complex landscape of hypothyroidism. This book aims to demystify the condition, offering clear, actionable steps to manage symptoms, optimize diet, and improve overall thyroid health.

Living with hypothyroidism can be an isolating experience, filled with frustration and unanswered questions. Many sufferers feel misunderstood or dismissed by the medical community, their symptoms downplayed as mere stress or aging. This book is here to validate your experiences and provide you with the tools to take control of your health.

The purpose of this book extends beyond merely providing information. It seeks to empower you with knowledge and practical strategies to reclaim your vitality and improve your quality of life. By understanding the underlying causes of hypothyroidism and the various treatment options available, you can make informed decisions and advocate effectively for your health.

Hypothyroidism requires a multifaceted approach to treatment and management. It's not just about taking medication; it's about adopting a holistic lifestyle that supports your thyroid function and overall well-being. This book will guide you through dietary changes, stress management techniques, and other lifestyle adjustments that can make a significant differ-ence in your health.

Why This Book is Different

What sets this book apart is its holistic approach and emphasis on actionable steps. Many books on hypothyroidism provide a wealth of information but fall short of practical advice. "Hypothyroidism Treatment Revolution" bridges this gap by offering clear, step-by-step guidance that you can implement immediately.

The strategies presented are backed by the latest research and clinical practices, but they are also grounded in real-world experience. Having lived with hypothyroidism for over two decades, I understand the day-to-day challenges and the importance of finding practical solutions that fit into a busy life.

Additionally, this book addresses the emotional and psycho-logical aspects of living with hypothyroidism. Chronic illness can take a toll on mental health, and it's essential to approach treatment with a holistic mindset that considers the whole person, not just the symptoms.

One of the central themes of this book is empowerment through action. Hypothyroidism can make you feel powerless, but by taking proactive steps, you can regain control over your health. Here are some initial actionable steps to get started:

1. Educate Yourself: Knowledge is power. The more you understand about hypothyroidism, the better equipped you will be to manage it. Use this book as a starting point and continue to seek out reputable sources of information.

2. Seek Support: Connect with others who are going through similar experiences. Support groups, both online and offline, can provide valuable emotional support and practical advice.

3. Monitor Your Symptoms: Keep a detailed journal of your symptoms, diet, and lifestyle habits. This can help you and your healthcare provider identify patterns and make more informed decisions about your treatment.

4. Advocate for Your Health: Don't be afraid to ask questions and seek second opinions. Your health is your most valuable asset, and it's important to find healthcare providers who listen to your concerns and work with you to develop a personalized treatment plan.

5. Make Lifestyle Changes: Small, consistent changes in diet, exercise, and stress management can have a significant impact on your thyroid health. Start with manageable goals and build from there.

6. Stay Positive and Patient: Managing hypothyroidism is a journey, not a destination. There will be ups and downs, but

with perseverance and the right strategies, you can improve your health and quality of life.

Understanding Your Body

Hypothyroidism affects everyone differently, and understanding your unique body is crucial to managing the condition effectively. Pay attention to how your body responds to different treatments, foods, and activities. This self-awareness will help you make informed choices that are best suited to your individual needs.

Isolation can be one of the most challenging aspects of living with hypothyroidism. Building a strong support network of friends, family, and fellow thyroid patients can provide emotional support and practical advice. Don't hesitate to reach out and share your journey with others who understand what you're going through.

Hypothyroidism is often a lifelong condition, and managing it requires a long-term commitment. This book will provide you with strategies for long-term management, helping you to stay on track and make sustainable changes that support your health over the years.

As you embark on this journey, keep an open mind, be patient with yourself, and stay committed to making positive changes. Your health and well-being are worth the effort. Let this book be your companion and guide as you navigate the path to better thyroid health.

This book is more than just a guide; it's a call to action. It's an invitation to take charge of your health and transform your life. By understanding your condition and implementing the strategies outlined, you can move from merely surviving to truly thriving.

Remember, you are not alone in this journey. Millions of people worldwide are living with hypothyroidism, and many have found ways to manage their symptoms and lead fulfilling lives. With the right tools and support, you can too.

As you embark on this journey, keep an open mind, be patient with yourself, and stay committed to making positive changes. Your health and well-being are worth the effort. Let this book be your companion and guide as you navigate the path to better thyroid health.

1

Understanding Hypothyroidism

"In its essence, the thyroid gland is the body's metronome, setting the rhythm for a myriad of metabolic processes that sustain life."

This statement by endocrinologist Dr. Terry Davies encapsulates the critical role of the thyroid gland in our overall health. Despite its small size, the thyroid gland's influence is vast, affecting virtually every cell, tissue, and organ in the body. According to the American Thyroid Association, an estimated 20 million Americans have some form of thyroid disease, and up to 60% of those with thyroid disease are unaware of their condition. This chapter delves into the complex world of hypothyroidism, a condition where the thyroid gland underperforms, leading to a cascade of health issues.

Understanding hypothyroidism begins with a clear definition and recognition of its various types. We explore the foundational concepts that underpin thyroid function and the hormonal interplay essential for maintaining metabolic balance. The subsequent sections illuminate the primary causes and risk factors associated with hypothyroidism, including autoimmune diseases like Hashimoto's thyroiditis and other influential factors such as medications and radiation exposure.

In this chapter, we also unravel the intricate mechanisms of the thyroid gland itself—how it produces crucial hormones like thyroxine (T4) and triiodothyronine (T3), and how these hormones regulate vital bodily functions. By gaining a comprehensive understanding of how the thyroid works, readers will be better equipped to recognize the significance of thyroid health and the impact of hypothyroidism on overall well-being. This journey through the fundamentals of hypothyroidism is designed to provide not just knowledge, but actionable insights to empower individuals in managing their health effectively.

1.1. What is Hypothyroidism

Hypothyroidism, also referred to as underactive thyroid disease, is a condition characterized by insufficient production of thyroid hormones by the thyroid gland to adequately meet the body's requirements. When there is a deficiency, it can cause various physiological and psychological effects since thyroid hormones are essential for regulating metabolism, energy production, and overall cellular function. Exploring hypothyroidism requires a deep dive into its definition, fundamental concepts, and the different types that exist.

Definition and Basic Concepts

The thyroid gland is a small, butterfly-shaped gland situated at the base of the neck, slightly below the Adam's apple. With its small stature, it manages to exert a profound influence on almost every cell in the body by secreting hormones, specifically thyroxine (T4) and triiodothyronine (T3). Hormones play a crucial role in regulating the body's metabolic rate, heart and digestive functions, muscle control, brain development, and bone maintenance.

When the thyroid gland fails to produce sufficient hormones, hypothyroidism can develop. This insufficiency can arise from a range of underlying causes, which will be explored in subsequent sections. When thyroid hormones are insufficient, the body's metabolic processes are affected, resulting in symptoms like fatigue, weight gain, cold intolerance, depression, and cognitive impairment.

In order to comprehend hypothyroidism, it is important to have a firm grasp on the feedback loop that involves the hypothalamus, pituitary gland, and thyroid gland. This axis, which serves a key role in maintaining thyroid hormone levels, is responsible for regulating the production and release of thyroid hormones. The hypothalamus releases a hormone called thyrotropin-releasing hormone (TRH), which then stimulates the pituitary gland to secrete thyroid-stimulating hormone (TSH). TSH stimulates the thyroid gland to produce T4 and T3. When the levels of these hormones are adequate, they send a signal to the hypothalamus and pituitary gland to decrease the release of TRH and TSH, thus ensuring a balanced hormonal state.

When there is an imbalance in hypothyroidism, the levels of TSH increase as the pituitary gland tries to stimulate the thyroid gland to produce more hormones. Even with all these efforts, the thyroid gland may still struggle to produce enough T4 and T3, leading to the typical symptoms of hypothyroidism.

Types of Hypothyroidism

There are various classifications of hypothyroidism, which are based on the causes and the specific part of the thyroid hormone production pathway that is impacted. There are several types of hypothyroidism, including primary, secondary, tertiary, congenital, and subclinical hypothyroidism.

Primary Hypothyroidism

The most common form of hypothyroidism is primary, which occurs when there is dysfunction in the thyroid gland itself. This type is commonly caused by autoimmune diseases, such as Hashimoto's thyroiditis, where the immune system mistakenly attacks the thyroid gland. Additional factors that can contribute to primary hypothyroidism are iodine deficiency, specific medications, radiation therapy, and surgical removal of the thyroid gland.

Hashimoto's Thyroiditis

Hashimoto's thyroiditis is an autoimmune disorder and the most common cause of hypothyroidism in areas with adequate iodine levels. With this condition, the immune system generates antibodies that specifically attack the thyroid gland, resulting in persistent inflammation and gradual deterioration of thyroid tissue. When the gland is damaged, its ability to produce thyroid hormones decreases, leading to hypothyroidism.

Individuals diagnosed with Hashimoto's thyroiditis commonly experience a goiter, along with symptoms like fatigue, weight gain, cold intolerance, constipation, dry skin, and depression. Diagnosis is confirmed by conducting blood tests to measure levels of TSH, T4, and T3, as well as the presence of thyroid antibodies such as anti-thyroid peroxidase (anti-TPO) and anti-thyroglobulin (anti-Tg).

Secondary and Tertiary Hypothyroidism

Secondary hypothyroidism occurs when the pituitary gland does not produce sufficient TSH to stimulate the thyroid gland. These occurrences may be a result of pituitary tumors, surgical procedures, radiation therapy, or traumatic brain injury. Given the interplay between the pituitary gland and the thyroid gland, any issues with the former can result in inadequate production of thyroid hormones.

Tertiary hypothyroidism is an extremely uncommon condition that arises when the hypothalamus does not generate sufficient TRH to prompt the pituitary gland to secrete TSH. This form of hypothyroidism may arise due to hypothalamic damage caused by factors such as tumors, trauma, or radiation therapy. The hypothalamus helps in regulating various important functions of the body. However, if its ability to release TRH is compromised, it can lead to a decrease in the production of thyroid hormones.

Congenital Hypothyroidism

Congenital hypothyroidism is a condition that is present at birth and can be caused by various factors, such as genetic mutations, developmental issues in the thyroid gland, or a lack of iodine during pregnancy. If left untreated, this condition can result in significant developmental problems. Early detection through newborn screening programs has played a vital role in preventing intellectual disability and growth failure in affected infants.

There are several genetic mutations that can lead to congenital hypothyroidism, impacting the development of the thyroid or the synthesis of hormones. In certain instances, the thyroid gland can be entirely absent, underdeveloped, or situated in an abnormal position. Genetic testing is valuable in identifying the specific mutations and providing guidance for treatment decisions.

Subclinical Hypothyroidism

Subclinical hypothyroidism is a mild form characterized by elevated TSH levels in the blood, while T4 and T3 levels remain within the normal range. It can be difficult to detect as it often doesn't present with obvious symptoms, and is usually identified through routine blood tests. For individuals with subclinical hypothyroidism, it may not be necessary to start treatment right away. However, it is important to regularly monitor and reassess the condition. With the passage of time, subclinical hypothyroidism has the potential to develop into overt hypothyroidism, where the symptoms become increasingly noticeable and the necessity for treatment becomes more pressing.

Subclinical hypothyroidism is quite prevalent among older adults and women, particularly those with a family history of thyroid disease. Various factors, including pregnancy, iodine intake, and specific medications, can impact the development of subclinical hypothyroidism into overt hypothyroidism. There is some variation in clinical guidelines regarding the treatment of subclinical hypothyroidism. However, treatment is typically recommended for individuals who exhibit symptoms, have a TSH level above 10 mIU/L, or have specific risk factors like pregnancy or cardiovascular disease.

1.2. Causes and Risk Factors

Hypothyroidism is a condition where the thyroid gland doesn't produce enough thyroid hormones. It can be caused by a variety of factors and risk factors. Having a deep understanding of these underlying factors is essential for accurately diagnosing, treating, and managing the condition. This section delves into the primary causes and risk factors linked to hypothyroidism, with a specific focus on autoimmune diseases like Hashimoto's thyroiditis, as well as other causes such as medications, radiation, and lifestyle factors.

Autoimmune Diseases

Autoimmune thyroiditis, specifically Hashimoto's thyroiditis, is a frequent culprit behind hypothyroidism. This condition occurs when the immune system mistakenly attacks the thyroid gland, resulting in inflammation and gradual destruction of thyroid tissue. The precise etiology of autoimmune thyroiditis remains somewhat elusive, although it is thought to encompass a complex interplay of genetic, environmental, and immunological elements.

Hashimoto's Thyroiditis

Hashimoto's thyroiditis, also referred to as chronic lymphocytic thyroiditis, is the most common type of autoimmune thyroiditis and is responsible for causing hypothyroidism in regions with adequate iodine levels. In Hashimoto's thyroiditis, the immune system generates antibodies that specifically attack thyroid proteins, including thyroid peroxidase (TPO) and thyroglobulin (Tg). These antibodies result in persistent inflammation and harm to the thyroid gland, which hinders its capacity to generate thyroid hormones.

Individuals diagnosed with Hashimoto's thyroiditis commonly encounter a gradual emergence of symptoms, which encompass fatigue, weight gain, cold intolerance, constipation, dry skin, and depression. It is worth noting that the condition is more prevalent among women compared to men, typically manifesting between the ages of 30 and 50. Having a family history of autoimmune diseases raises the likelihood of developing Hashimoto's thyroiditis, indicating a genetic predisposition.

Exploring Other Autoimmune Diseases

Other autoimmune diseases can also play a role in the development of hypothyroidism, alongside Hashimoto's thyroiditis. Medical conditions like type 1 diabetes, rheumatoid arthritis, lupus, and Addison's disease have been found to be linked with a higher likelihood of developing hypothyroidism. Having one autoimmune disease can raise the chances of developing another, since the immune system dysfunction that underlies it affects various organs and systems.

Other Possible Factors

Although autoimmune thyroiditis is a common cause of hypothyroidism, there are various other factors that can also play a role in the development of this condition. These options encompass a range of treatments, such as medications, radiation therapy, surgical procedures, and various lifestyle and environmental factors.

Prescription drugs

Some medications can disrupt the production or function of thyroid hormones, resulting in hypothyroidism. Some medications can potentially lead to hypothyroidism:

1. 1. Amiodarone: This antiarrhythmic medication is commonly prescribed to address irregular heart rhythms. It is important to note that due to its high iodine content, amiodarone has the potential to interfere with the synthesis of thyroid hormones, potentially resulting in hypothyroidism.
2. 2. Lithium is commonly prescribed to manage bipolar

disorder. However, it's important to note that this medication can have an impact on thyroid hormone release, potentially resulting in hypothyroidism.

3. Interferon-alpha is commonly prescribed for the treatment of hepatitis C and certain cancers. However, it is important to note that this medication can potentially lead to the development of autoimmune thyroiditis and hypothyroidism.

4. Tyrosine kinase inhibitors can lead to thyroid dysfunction as they hinder the thyroid gland's hormone production.

It is important for individuals on these medications to undergo regular thyroid function monitoring in order to promptly identify and address any potential hypothyroidism.

Radiation therapy

When radiation therapy is used to treat cancers of the head, neck, and chest, it can have a negative impact on the thyroid gland, leading to a decrease in hormone production. This form of hypothyroidism may manifest months or even years following exposure to radiation. Radioactive iodine treatment is commonly used to address hyperthyroidism or thyroid cancer. However, it's important to note that this treatment can also result in hypothyroidism due to the destruction of thyroid tissue.

Regular follow-up and thyroid function tests are necessary for patients with radiation-induced hypothyroidism to detect the onset of the condition and start hormone replacement therapy as needed. When dealing with this form of hypothyroidism, it is important to find a balance between the advantages of cancer treatment and the necessity of preserving thyroid health.

Medical Procedures

Thyroid surgery, such as thyroidectomy or lobectomy, may lead to hypothyroidism. Surgeries like these are commonly done to address thyroid cancer, noncancerous thyroid nodules, or hyperthyroidism. After the removal of a significant portion of the thyroid gland, the remaining tissue might struggle to produce sufficient hormone levels, resulting in hypothyroidism.

Patients who undergo thyroidectomy or lobectomy usually need to take thyroid hormone replacement therapy for the rest of their lives to keep their metabolic function in check. Consistent monitoring of TSH and thyroid hormone levels is crucial for dosage adjustments and to ensure effective management.

Iodine deficiency

Iodine plays a crucial role in the production of thyroid hormones. Insufficient iodine intake may result in hypothyroidism as the thyroid gland is unable to produce adequate hormones without it. Iodine deficiency continues to be a major concern for public health in numerous regions across the globe, especially in areas where iodine is not fortified in table salt or food.

Common signs of hypothyroidism caused by iodine deficiency include an enlarged thyroid gland (goiter), fatigue, weight gain, and cognitive impairment. Implementing preventive measures, such as incorporating iodized salt and dietary supplements, has proven to be highly effective in decreasing the occurrence of iodine deficiency and related thyroid disorders.

Environmental factors

Certain chemicals and pollutants in the environment can also affect thyroid function and contribute to hypothyroidism. It is worth noting that perchlorate, a chemical commonly found in rocket fuel, explosives, and certain fertilizers, has the potential to disrupt the thyroid gland's capacity to absorb iodine. Various environmental toxins, like polychlorinated biphenyls (PCBs) and bisphenol A (BPA), have the potential to interfere with endocrine function and impact the production of thyroid hormones.

Risk Factors

There are several factors that can increase the chances of developing hypothyroidism. These factors encompass genetic predisposition, age, gender, and specific medical conditions and treatments.

Genetic Predisposition

Having a family history of thyroid disease or autoimmune conditions can raise the chances of developing hypothyroidism. Genetic factors have a substantial impact on the onset of autoimmune thyroiditis, including Hashimoto's thyroiditis. There are certain genes that can make individuals more susceptible to autoimmune thyroid disease, as they are involved in regulating the immune system and thyroid function.

Age and gender

Hypothyroidism is more prevalent in women compared to men and tends to become more frequent as individuals age. During periods of hormonal change, such as pregnancy, postpartum, and menopause, women are more prone to developing hypothyroidism. As individuals grow older, their likelihood of developing hypothyroidism increases, making older adults more susceptible to this condition.

Medical Conditions

Some medical conditions have a higher likelihood of being linked to hypothyroidism. Here are some examples:

1. Type 1 Diabetes: An autoimmune condition that may contribute to the development of autoimmune thyroiditis and hypothyroidism.

2. Rheumatoid Arthritis is another autoimmune disorder that can coexist with autoimmune thyroid disease.

3. Lupus is a systemic autoimmune disease that has the potential to impact various organs, including the thyroid gland.

4. Addison's Disease is an autoimmune condition that affects the adrenal glands and can be linked to hypothyroidism.

Factors that can influence one's lifestyle

Various lifestyle factors, including dietary choices and stress levels, have the potential to impact thyroid function and play a role in the development of hypothyroidism. A diet lacking in vital nutrients, such as iodine, selenium, and zinc, can hinder the production of thyroid hormones. Chronic stress has the potential to impact the HPT axis, which can disrupt the regular regulation of thyroid hormone production.

1.3. How the Thyroid Works

The thyroid gland, commonly referred to as a butterfly-shaped organ located at the base of the neck, may seem small and unassuming at first sight. However, its influence on the human body is extensive and significant. This gland plays a crucial role in producing and releasing hormones that help regulate the body's metabolism, growth, and development. Having a good grasp of the function and hormones of the thyroid is essential for understanding how this gland impacts overall health.

Thyroid Hormones: The Key Players

Thyroxine (T4) and triiodothyronine (T3) are the two primary hormones produced by the thyroid gland. Both of these hormones play a crucial role in regulating the body's metabolic rate, which determines how quickly the body converts food into energy.

Thyroxine (T4)

Thyroxine, also known as T4, is the predominant hormone produced by the thyroid gland, making up around 90% of the hormones released. The hormone contains four iodine atoms, which is evident from its name. Although T4 is produced in larger quantities, it is relatively less active compared to T3. It functions as a pro-hormone, with its main purpose being to act as a precursor to T3. After being released into the bloodstream, T4 travels to different tissues and undergoes conversion into the more potent T3 hormone. This conversion process mainly occurs in the liver and kidneys, as well as other tissues, to ensure that T3 is readily available in the areas where it is most necessary.

Triiodothyronine (T3)

T3 is considered to be the strongest of the two thyroid hormones. This compound has three iodine atoms and is much more potent than T4. Despite the fact that only a small percentage of the thyroid hormones released by the gland are T3, this particular hormone is responsible for the majority of the biological effects associated with thyroid hormones. T3 has a significant impact on numerous metabolic processes, affecting a wide range of cells throughout the body. It interacts with thyroid hormone receptors in the cell nuclei, triggering transcription and resulting in the synthesis of proteins that control metabolism, growth, and development.

Production and Regulation: The HPT Axis

The production and release of thyroid hormones are carefully controlled by the HPT axis, which is a feedback loop that includes the hypothalamus, pituitary gland, and thyroid gland. This axis ensures that the body maintains optimal levels of thyroid hormones, adjusting production based on the body's needs.

The process starts in the hypothalamus, a small region of the brain that functions as the body's thermostat. When the hypothalamus detects low levels of thyroid hormones in the blood, it releases thyrotropin-releasing hormone (TRH). TRH makes its way to the pituitary gland, a vital gland situated at the base of the brain. When TRH is detected, the pituitary gland releases thyroid-stimulating hormone (TSH) into the bloodstream. TSH then travels to the thyroid gland, prompting the production and release of T4 and T3.

When T4 and T3 levels increase in the bloodstream, they send negative feedback signals to the hypothalamus and pituitary gland. This feedback mechanism helps regulate the release of

TRH and TSH, which prevents excessive production of thyroid hormones and keeps the hormonal balance in check.

The Biological Impact of Thyroid Hormones

Thyroid hormones are essential for regulating metabolism, encompassing all the chemical reactions necessary to sustain life within the body. Hormones have a significant impact on the basal metabolic rate (BMR), which is the amount of energy the body uses while at rest. Thyroid hormones play a vital role in boosting the body's calorie-burning efficiency, resulting in a higher metabolic rate. This is why weight gain and a decrease in metabolic rate are commonly observed in individuals with hypothyroidism.

Thyroid hormones also increase the body's responsiveness to catecholamines, hormones produced by the adrenal glands, like adrenaline. This mechanism enhances heart rate and cardiac output, effectively facilitating the delivery of oxygen and nutrients to tissues and organs. Individuals with hypothyroidism commonly experience a slower heart rate and reduced circulation, which can lead to symptoms such as fatigue and cold extremities.

Thyroid hormones play an essential role in growth and development, especially in children, in addition to their metabolic functions. They promote protein synthesis, bone growth, and the maturation of the nervous system. Early detection and treatment of thyroid disorders in young individuals is important as inadequate levels of thyroid hormones during childhood can result in growth retardation and cognitive impairments.

Thermogenesis and Heat Production

Thyroid hormones support thermogenesis, which is the body's way of generating heat. Thyroid hormones have a key role in regulating the body's internal temperature by boosting the metabolic rate, which helps generate heat and maintain stability. Individuals with hypothyroidism often experience feelings of coldness and struggle to maintain body warmth due to their reduced hormone levels, which result in a decreased ability to produce heat.

Effects on the Digestive System

Thyroid hormones have a significant impact on the digestive system. They enhance the production of digestive enzymes and facilitate the smooth movement of food through the digestive tract. When thyroid hormone levels are low in the body, digestion can be affected, resulting in symptoms like constipation and bloating. By ensuring optimal thyroid hormone levels, the digestive system operates more efficiently, promoting proper nutrient absorption and waste elimination.

Neurological and Cognitive Functions

The impact of thyroid hormones reaches the brain and nervous system. Thyroid hormones help in the development of the brain and cognitive function during fetal development and early childhood. They play a crucial role in promoting the formation of myelin, the fatty substance that envelops nerve fibers and aids in the smooth transmission of nerve impulses. Having optimal thyroid hormone levels is essential for cognitive function, memory retention, and overall psychological well-being.

Thyroid hormones assist in maintaining cognitive function and mood in adults. Cognitive impairments, such as difficulty concentrating, memory problems, and depression, can be associated with hypothyroidism. These symptoms, commonly known as "brain fog," can have a significant impact on one's daily life. Ensuring proper thyroid hormone levels is crucial for maintaining optimal brain function and emotional well-being.

Exploring the Impact on the Musculoskeletal System

The musculoskeletal system relies on thyroid hormones for its development and maintenance. They have a big role in bone remodeling, a constant process of replacing old bone tissue with new bone tissue. This process is absolutely vital for preserving bone strength and density. Thyroid hormones have a big impact in ensuring proper bone growth and development in children. Insufficient levels of thyroid hormone during childhood may result in stunted growth and delayed development of the skeletal system.

Thyroid hormones play a crucial role in preserving muscle mass and strength in adults. They help promote protein synthesis, which is essential for the repair and growth of muscles. Individuals with hypothyroidism may experience symptoms such as muscle weakness, cramps, and joint pain. These symptoms can arise from reduced protein synthesis and impaired muscle function. Ensuring optimal thyroid hormone levels is crucial for maintaining musculoskeletal health and enhancing physical performance.

Reproductive Health

Thyroid hormones also have an impact on reproductive health. They perform a crucial role in regulating menstrual cycles and supporting fertility in women. Menstrual irregularities, such as heavy or irregular periods, can be a result of hypothyroidism. Additionally, hypothyroidism can impact ovulation, making it more difficult to conceive. In men, thyroid hormones support testosterone production and the regulation of sperm production. Men with hypothyroidism may experience a decrease in sexual desire, difficulties with achieving or maintaining an erection, and potential issues with fertility. Ensuring the right balance of thyroid hormones is key for promoting reproductive health and overall well-being.

Skin, Hair, and Nails

Thyroid hormones have a significant impact on the skin, hair, and nails. They enhance cell turnover and stimulate the production of collagen, a vital protein that contributes to the skin's structure and resilience. Having optimal thyroid hormone levels is crucial for the well-being of your skin, hair, and nails. Individuals with hypothyroidism may experience symptoms such as dry, rough skin, brittle hair, and weak nails. These manifestations are a result of reduced cell turnover and collagen production. Hair loss is a frequently observed symptom of hypothyroidism, since thyroid hormones have an impact on the hair growth cycle. Keeping thyroid hormone levels in check is important for promoting the well-being and overall look of the skin, hair, and nails.

Conclusion

As we conclude our exploration of hypothyroidism, it is evident that the thyroid gland, despite its modest size, plays an indispensable role in maintaining our health. Hypothyroidism, characterized by insufficient production of thyroid hormones, can lead to widespread physiological disruptions, affecting metabolism, cardiovascular health, digestion, musculoskeletal integrity, neurological function, and reproductive health.

Recognizing the symptoms and understanding the underlying causes of hypothyroidism is the first step toward effective management and treatment.

This chapter has highlighted the fundamental aspects of thyroid function, the production and regulation of thyroid hormones, and the extensive impact these hormones have on the body. By examining the various types of hypothyroidism, from autoimmune thyroiditis to environmentally induced thyroid dysfunction, we gain a deeper appreciation for the complexity of this condition. The insights provided here aim to equip you with the knowledge to identify potential thyroid issues early and seek appropriate medical intervention.

In the chapters that follow, we will delve deeper into the symptoms of hypothyroidism, diagnostic procedures, and the array of treatment options available. By continuing this journey, you will be better prepared to manage hypothyroidism effectively, improve your quality of life, and maintain optimal health. The knowledge gained in this chapter lays the foundation for a comprehensive approach to understanding and living with hypothyroidism.

2

Symptoms of Hypothyroidism

"Symptoms are the body's language, speaking to us in signs and sensations."

This quote by unknown but profound author reminds us that our bodies often communicate their needs and distress through various symptoms. Hypothyroidism, a condition characterized by an underactive thyroid gland, is no exception. According to the American Thyroid Association, approximately 12% of the U.S. population will develop a thyroid condition during their lifetime, with hypothyroidism being one of the most common. Despite its prevalence, many people remain undiagnosed, largely due to the subtle and varied nature of its symptoms.

This chapter delves into the myriad symptoms associated with hypothyroidism, offering a detailed exploration of both physical and cognitive-emotional manifestations. Understanding these symptoms is crucial for early diagnosis and effective management. From relentless fatigue and unexplained weight gain to depression and cognitive decline, the symptoms of

30

hypothyroidism can significantly impair one's quality of life. By recognizing these signs and seeking timely medical evaluation, individuals can take proactive steps toward restoring their health and well-being.

We will begin by examining the common physical symptoms, shedding light on how hypothyroidism affects various bodily functions. Following this, we will explore the cognitive and emotional symptoms that often accompany the condition, providing insights into how hypothyroidism impacts mental health. Finally, we will discuss the diagnostic process, high-lighting the importance of comprehensive medical history, physical examination, and laboratory tests in confirming the presence of hypothyroidism. Through this comprehensive overview, we aim to equip readers with the knowledge and tools needed to identify and manage hypothyroidism effectively.

2.1. Common Symptoms

Manifesting through a range of symptoms, hypothyroidism is a condition that often goes unnoticed and can have a profound impact on one's quality of life. These symptoms can be divided into two main categories: physical symptoms and cognitive and emotional symptoms. Recognizing and understanding these symptoms is essential for early diagnosis and effective management of hypothyroidism.

Physical Symptoms

Hypothyroidism can be compared to a stealthy intruder that silently infiltrates different bodily systems, causing disruptions to normal function. The physical manifestations of this condition can have a wide-ranging impact, influencing various aspects such as energy levels and skin health. Gaining a thorough understanding of these symptoms not only helps with diagnosis, but also emphasizes the significant influence that thyroid health has on one's overall well-being.

Fatigue and Weakness

Fatigue is a commonly experienced symptom of hypothyroidism. This fatigue goes beyond the usual tiredness and persists despite attempts to rest and recharge. Picture waking up with the sensation of having completed a strenuous workout while you were asleep, your muscles feeling weighed down and your drive depleted. This constant fatigue is a result of the vital role that thyroid hormones play in controlling the body's metabolism. When these hormones are lacking, the body's cells do not receive sufficient energy to function effectively, resulting in a constant state of fatigue and debility. Everyday activities can feel overwhelming, and even getting out of bed can seem impossible.

Weight Gain and Difficulty Losing Weight

Weight gain in hypothyroidism is not solely caused by overeating or lack of exercise; rather, it is a direct outcome of a slowed metabolism. Thyroid hormones help regulate metabolic rate, which determines how quickly the body can burn calories. When hormone levels decrease, the metabolic rate also decreases, resulting in the body storing more calories as fat. This can occur even if an individual's diet and physical activity levels remain constant. In addition, hypothyroidism can cause fluid retention, which can worsen weight gain. For many people, the challenge lies in the struggle to shed those extra pounds, as the body's ability to burn fat is greatly hindered.

Cold Intolerance

Feeling cold constantly, even in warm environments, is a common symptom of hypothyroidism. This cold intolerance occurs because thyroid hormones support the body's thermogenesis process, which involves heat production. When hormone levels are low, the body's ability to generate and retain heat is compromised. These symptoms often result in a sensation of coldness in the hands and feet, as well as a reduced ability to tolerate cooler temperatures. For certain individuals, this symptom can be incredibly debilitating, affecting their everyday activities and requiring them to wear multiple layers of clothing or rely on extra heating to maintain comfort.

Dry Skin and Hair

The health of skin and hair is intricately connected to thyroid function. Thyroid hormones play a crucial role in supporting cell turnover and collagen production, which are vital for keeping your skin smooth and your hair healthy and strong. With hypothyroidism, there is a decrease in hormone levels which results in a reduction of cell turnover and collagen production: the outcome is skin that becomes dry, rough, and flaky. Hair can become rough, fragile, and more likely to fall out. Thinning of the eyebrows, especially on the outer edges, can be a clear indication of thyroid dysfunction. These changes can be quite distressing, impacting one's self-esteem and overall appearance.

Constipation

Many individuals with hypothyroidism often experience digestive issues, including constipation. Thyroid hormones help regulate the motility of the digestive tract, ensuring the smooth movement of food and waste through the intestines. When hormone levels decrease, the motility of the digestive system slows down, resulting in constipation. This symptom can be quite uncomfortable and can pose a challenge to manage. It often necessitates dietary adjustments and occasionally medication to provide relief.

Muscle Weakness and Joint Pain

People with hypothyroidism often experience muscle and joint problems. Individuals may experience muscle weakness, cramps, and joint pain as a result of reduced protein synthesis and compromised muscle repair and maintenance. Experiencing stiff, aching joints upon waking or feeling muscle fatigue with minimal exertion are quite common occurrences. These symptoms can be physically limiting and also have an impact on one's emotional well-being, making daily activities more challenging and less enjoyable.

High Cholesterol Levels

Thyroid hormones are essential for lipid metabolism and play a vital role in regulating cholesterol levels within the body. When hormone levels decrease in hypothyroidism, it can result in higher levels of low-density lipoprotein (LDL) cholesterol, commonly known as "bad" cholesterol. This elevation in cholesterol levels can significantly increase the likelihood of developing serious cardiovascular conditions, including atherosclerosis, heart attacks, and strokes. It is crucial for individuals with hypothyroidism to regularly monitor and manage their cholesterol levels in order to prevent potential complications.

Menstrual Irregularities

Women with hypothyroidism may experience disruptions in their menstrual cycle, resulting in irregularities such as heavy or prolonged periods, irregular cycles, or missed periods. An imbalance in thyroid hormones can have an impact on the menstrual cycle, as they interact with reproductive hormones. These disruptions can also affect fertility, making it more difficult for women with hypothyroidism to become pregnant. Menstrual irregularities can cause a lot of stress and discomfort, which can really impact your overall quality of life.

Swelling in the Neck (Goiter)

There are instances where hypothyroidism can lead to the enlargement of the thyroid gland, which can then cause a goiter. This noticeable swelling in the neck occurs as the thyroid tries to compensate for its decreased hormone production by enlarging. When a goiter grows larger, it can lead to discomfort, trouble swallowing, or difficulties with breathing. However, in some cases, a goiter may not cause any pain and may only be a cosmetic issue. Having a goiter can serve as a physical sign of thyroid dysfunction, which usually leads to additional medical examinations.

Cognitive and Emotional Symptoms

Hypothyroidism, which is often overshadowed by its more visible physical symptoms, can have a significant impact on cognitive and emotional health. These symptoms can be difficult to detect, sneaky, and are often mistaken for other conditions, resulting in delays in diagnosis and treatment. Having a deep understanding of the cognitive and emotional impact of hypothyroidism is essential for effectively managing the condition.

Depression and Anxiety

Depression can be a significant emotional effect of hypothyroidism. This is not just occasional sadness; it is a pervasive sense of despair, fatigue, and disinterest in activities that once brought joy. Insufficient thyroid hormone production can lead to biochemical imbalances that impact neurotransmitter levels in the brain, including serotonin, a key player in mood regulation. When serotonin levels decrease, depressive symptoms increase, resulting in a constant sense of gloom and hopelessness.

Another emotional symptom that is frequently experienced is anxiety. People with hypothyroidism may experience persistent anxiety, restlessness, and a feeling of imminent danger. This heightened state of anxiety may arise from the body's challenge to operate at its best without adequate thyroid hormones, leading to an overactive stress response. When depression and anxiety come together, they can create a harmful cycle, where worry intensifies sadness, and vice versa, significantly affecting daily life.

Memory problems and Cognitive Decline

Brain fog is a common occurrence in hypothyroidism, characterized by cognitive symptoms. This term accurately captures the challenges people face when it comes to processing information, maintaining focus, and remembering things. Thyroid hormones help cognitive function, impacting brain development, synaptic plasticity, and neurogenesis. When these hormones are lacking, cognitive processes can become sluggish, resulting in memory lapses, difficulty focusing, and reduced mental clarity.

Individuals with hypothyroidism commonly report experiencing cognitive sluggishness. Everyday tasks that used to be easy now feel like a struggle, and it's harder to juggle multiple things at once. This decline in cognitive function can have a significant impact on one's professional performance, academic achievements, and daily responsibilities, leading to feelings of frustration and a decrease in self-esteem.

Slowed Speech and Movement

Psychomotor retardation, a common symptom of hypothyroidism, is characterized by slowed thought processes and physical movements. These symptoms can present themselves in different ways, including speech that is slower, response times that are delayed, and a decrease in physical activity. People may notice a decrease in their speaking speed and fluency, which can make conversations more difficult and less interesting.

This decrease in psychomotor activity also impacts physical movements. Tasks that involve precise hand movements, such as writing or typing, can become more challenging. Experiencing a decline in both mental and physical functions can make everyday activities incredibly tiring, resulting in a greater need for assistance and a diminished sense of self-reliance.

Decreased Libido

Reproductive hormones can be affected by hypothyroidism, leading to a decrease in libido. This symptom can impact individuals of all genders and may result in a decrease in sexual desire. When it comes to women, an imbalance of thyroid hormones can cause disruptions in the menstrual cycle, which can have an impact on ovulation and fertility. In men, hypothyroidism can result in decreased testosterone levels, which can contribute to issues such as erectile dysfunction and a decrease in sexual desire.

This decrease in sexual desire can put a strain on personal relationships and worsen feelings of sadness and worry. It is important for individuals experiencing these symptoms to have open communication with their partners and seek medical advice to address the underlying hormonal imbalances.

Irritability and Mood Swings

Emotional instability is a frequently disregarded symptom of hypothyroidism. People may go through unexpected changes in mood, transitioning from being easily annoyed to feeling down without any clear reason. Managing this level of emotional volatility can be quite challenging, as it has a significant impact on interpersonal relationships and daily interactions.

The irritability linked to hypothyroidism may arise from the frustration of managing persistent fatigue, cognitive impairment, and physical discomfort. This irritability can result in conflicts with family, friends, and colleagues, which can further isolate the individual and exacerbate depressive symptoms.

Social Withdrawal and Isolation

The combination of these symptoms often results in individuals isolating themselves from social interactions. People with hypothyroidism may start to avoid social situations, feeling too tired or overwhelmed to interact with others. This withdrawal can contribute to a sense of isolation, which can intensify feelings of loneliness and depression.

Having a strong network of social support is essential for maintaining good mental health, as the absence of such support can lead to significant negative outcomes. It is crucial to emphasize the significance of maintaining social connections for individuals with hypothyroidism, even when it may seem difficult. Support groups, whether they are held in person or online, can offer a valuable sense of community and empathy, which can help alleviate the sense of isolation.

2.2. Diagnosing Hypothyroidism

Diagnosing hypothyroidism is an essential step in effectively managing and treating this condition. Accurate diagnosis is crucial for initiating appropriate therapies to restore normal thyroid function and alleviate the various symptoms associated with hypothyroidism. This section explores the comprehensive procedure for diagnosing hypothyroidism, covering important elements such as medical history, physical examination, and a range of diagnostic tests.

Medical History and Physical Exam

Diagnosing hypothyroidism typically starts with a comprehensive medical history. Understanding the patient's symptoms, lifestyle, and potential risk factors is important for healthcare providers to provide comprehensive care.

During the initial consultation, the healthcare provider will inquire about the patient's symptoms in great detail. It's crucial to address all symptoms, even if they may not appear to be connected, since hypothyroidism can have various manifestations. Common questions may involve symptoms such as fatigue, weight gain, cold intolerance, constipation, dry skin, hair loss, and menstrual irregularities. Depression, anxiety, memory problems, and irritability are also relevant cognitive and emotional symptoms.

Aside from symptomatology, the medical history will encompass other factors like the patient's family history of thyroid or autoimmune diseases, their past medical history which includes any previous thyroid disorders, surgeries, or radiation treatments to the neck, as well as any medications or supplements they are currently taking. It is important to disclose certain medications, such as lithium and amiodarone, as they can have an impact on thyroid function.

Gaining insights into the patient's lifestyle can be incredibly valuable. Various factors, such as dietary habits, exposure to environmental toxins, and stress levels, can have an impact on thyroid health. As an expert in the field, it's important to note that maintaining proper iodine intake is essential for the production of thyroid hormones. Imbalances in iodine levels, whether too little or too much, can result in thyroid dysfunction.

Performing a Physical Examination

After reviewing the medical history, a thorough physical examination is conducted to identify any physical indicators of hypothyroidism. A healthcare provider will examine the thyroid gland by feeling it for any signs of enlargement, nodules, or tenderness. Having an enlarged thyroid can be a sign of various thyroid disorders, such as hypothyroidism caused by Hashimoto's thyroiditis.

Additional physical indications that can be noticed include parched, rough skin, fragile hair, and a reduction in the density of the eyebrows' outer edges. As part of the examination, the healthcare professional will also look for any indications of fluid retention, such as swelling in the face, hands, and feet. They will also evaluate the heart rate, as a slower than normal heart rate, known as bradycardia, can be a possible sign of hypothyroidism.

Diagnostic Procedures and Blood Tests

Although the medical history and physical exam are important, laboratory tests are essential for accurately diagnosing hypothyroidism. These tests assess different parameters to assess thyroid function and determine the root cause of thyroid dysfunction.

Thyroid-Stimulating Hormone (TSH) Test

The TSH test serves as the main screening tool for hypothyroidism. TSH is produced by the pituitary gland and it plays a crucial role in stimulating the thyroid gland to produce thyroid hormones (T4 and T3). In cases of hypothyroidism, the thyroid gland does not produce enough hormones, causing an increase in TSH levels as the pituitary gland tries to make up for it.

High TSH levels are usually a sign of primary hypothyroidism, indicating that the issue originates from the thyroid gland itself. On the other hand, if someone experiences hypothyroid symptoms despite having low or normal TSH levels, it could indicate secondary or tertiary hypothyroidism. In these cases, the dysfunction originates in the pituitary gland or hypothalamus, respectively.

Free Thyroxine (Free T4) Test

Measuring levels of free thyroxine (T4) can offer valuable insights into thyroid function. Free T4 is the portion of T4 in the blood that is not bound and can be taken up by tissues. In cases of hypothyroidism, free T4 levels tend to be low, indicating that the thyroid gland is not able to produce sufficient hormone levels. This test is useful for confirming the diagnosis and evaluating the extent of hypothyroidism.

Free Triiodothyronine (Free T3) Test

While T4 is the main hormone produced by the thyroid gland, T3 is considered to be the more active form. Measuring free T3 levels can offer valuable insights, especially when T4 and TSH levels do not provide a clear picture. Free T3 levels in hypothyroidism can vary, either being low or falling within the normal range. This variation is influenced by the stage and severity of the condition.

Thyroid Antibody Tests

Autoimmune thyroiditis, specifically Hashimoto's thyroiditis, is a prevalent cause of hypothyroidism. Thyroid antibody tests, such as anti-thyroid peroxidase (anti-TPO) and anti-thyroglobulin (anti-Tg) antibodies, are useful in identifying autoimmune thyroid disease. High levels of these antibodies suggest an autoimmune reaction against the thyroid gland, confirming Hashimoto's thyroiditis as the root cause of hypothyroidism.

Thyroid Ultrasound

Thyroid ultrasounds are sometimes conducted to provide a visual representation of the thyroid gland's structure. This imaging test is capable of identifying nodules, cysts, or an enlarged thyroid. Ultrasound is highly valuable for assessing goiters and differentiating between various types of thyroid nodules. This procedure is non-invasive and offers detailed images of the thyroid gland, aiding in the guidance of additional diagnostic and therapeutic choices.

Radioactive Iodine Uptake Test

Similar to the work of an experienced endocrinologist, the RAIU test evaluates the thyroid gland's ability to absorb iodine, a crucial element for the production of thyroid hormones. During this procedure, a small quantity of radioactive iodine is consumed by the patient, and a specialized camera gauges the thyroid gland's iodine absorption. This test is useful for differentiating between various causes of hypothyroidism, including autoimmune thyroiditis, iodine deficiency, and thyroiditis caused by other factors.

Additional Diagnostic Tests

Additional tests may be necessary in certain situations to determine any underlying causes or related conditions. As an expert in endocrinology, I would like to highlight that lipid profiles can be ordered to evaluate cholesterol levels, as hypothyroidism commonly results in increased LDL cholesterol. Blood glucose tests may also be performed to screen for diabetes, which can occur alongside thyroid disorders. Anemia is a common finding in hypothyroidism, so a complete blood count (CBC) can be helpful in ruling it out.

Conclusion

As we conclude our exploration of the symptoms of hypothyroidism, it becomes evident that this condition manifests in a wide array of physical, cognitive, and emotional signs. From the pervasive fatigue and weight gain that disrupt daily life to the cognitive fog and mood disturbances that erode mental well-being, hypothyroidism's impact is far-reaching and profound. Recognizing these symptoms early is essential for obtaining a timely diagnosis and initiating effective treatment.

The physical symptoms, such as cold intolerance, dry skin, and constipation, are often the most noticeable but can be easily mistaken for other health issues. Similarly, the cognitive and emotional symptoms, including depression, anxiety, and memory problems, can significantly impair one's quality of life but are frequently misattributed to stress or aging. This chapter has underscored the importance of understanding the full spectrum of hypothyroidism symptoms and the need for a comprehensive approach to diagnosis.

Accurate diagnosis is the cornerstone of effective treatment. By combining a detailed medical history, thorough physical examination, and specific laboratory tests, healthcare providers can confirm the presence of hypothyroidism and identify its underlying cause. This holistic diagnostic approach ensures that patients receive personalized and effective care.

Understanding the symptoms of hypothyroidism is the first step toward reclaiming health and well-being. Armed with this knowledge, individuals can seek appropriate medical advice, adhere to prescribed treatments, and make informed lifestyle choices to manage their condition. As we move forward, the subsequent chapters will delve into the various treatment options and lifestyle modifications that can help manage hypothyroidism, offering hope and practical solutions for those affected by this common yet often overlooked condition.

3

Treatment Options

"Medicine is not only a science; it is also an art. It does not consist of compounding pills and plasters; it deals with the very processes of life."

This insightful quote by Paracelsus sets the stage for our exploration of the diverse treatment options available for managing hypothyroidism. Hypothyroidism, characterized by an underactive thyroid gland, affects millions of people worldwide, leading to symptoms like fatigue, weight gain, and cognitive decline. While conventional treatments such as thyroid hormone replacement therapy (THRT) are highly effective and widely used, many patients seek additional or alternative approaches to enhance their health and well-being.

This chapter delves into the multifaceted world of hypothyroidism treatment, exploring both conventional and alternative methods. We begin by examining the cornerstone of conventional treatment, THRT, focusing on the use of levothyroxine and other thyroid hormone preparations. We then transition to the critical aspect of medication management, highlighting the importance of personalized dosing and monitoring to optimize treatment outcomes.

Following the discussion on conventional treatments, we venture into the realm of alternative therapies. These natural and integrative treatments offer valuable support, especially for those who continue to experience symptoms despite standard medical care.

By understanding and incorporating both conventional and alternative treatments, individuals with hypothyroidism can achieve a more balanced and effective management of their condition. This holistic approach not only addresses the underlying thyroid dysfunction but also enhances overall health and quality of life, paving the way for a more empowered and informed journey towards optimal thyroid health.

3.1. Conventional Treatments

Treating hypothyroidism is a fundamental part of effectively managing the condition and enhancing the well-being of individuals impacted by it. Conventional treatments primarily aim to restore normal thyroid hormone levels, alleviate symptoms, and prevent complications. This section explores the fundamental aspect of traditional hypothyroidism treatment:

Thyroid Hormone Replacement Therapy, and the intricacies of medication management.

Thyroid Hormone Replacement Therapy

Thyroid Hormone Replacement Therapy (THRT) is widely recognized as the most effective treatment for hypothyroidism. The main objective of this treatment is to provide the body with artificial thyroid hormones, which help to balance hormone levels and relieve the symptoms of hypothyroidism. Levothyroxine is the most commonly prescribed medication for THRT.

Levothyroxine: The Cornerstone of THRT

Levothyroxine, a synthetic form of thyroxine (T4), is considered the foundation of Thyroid Hormone Replacement Therapy (THRT), highlighting its crucial role in the treatment of hypothyroidism. This medication, which is highly valued by individuals with an underactive thyroid, replicates the T4 hormone naturally produced by the thyroid gland. The introduction of this treatment has brought about a significant change in the way hypothyroidism is treated, providing a dependable and efficient method to restore normal thyroid function and enhance overall quality of life.

Levothyroxine is highly valued in THRT due to its remarkable stability and unwavering consistency. Levothyroxine offers a consistent and reliable dose of thyroid hormone, unlike certain medications that may have inconsistent potency or effectiveness. Consistency plays a vital role in keeping thyroid hormone levels stable in the bloodstream, ensuring proper regulation of metabolism, energy production, and overall bodily function. Patients generally take levothyroxine once daily, which makes it easier to stick to the treatment and seamlessly incorporate it into their daily routines.

Starting the levothyroxine journey involves a thorough evaluation of the initial dosage. Healthcare providers consider a range of factors when determining the best course of action for patients, such as their age, weight, the severity of hypothyroidism, and any other health conditions they may have. The objective is to initiate treatment with a dosage that achieves the desired outcome while minimizing any potential negative consequences. For many individuals, it is common to start with a lower dose and make gradual adjustments based on the patient's response and regular blood tests.

Consistent monitoring is an essential aspect of successful levothyroxine treatment. At first, patients are required to have blood tests every 6 to 8 weeks in order to measure the levels of Thyroid-Stimulating Hormone (TSH) and free T4. These tests can assist in determining if any adjustments to the dosage are necessary. Once the optimal dose is determined, the frequency of monitoring may decrease, but it is still important to periodically test to ensure effectiveness and make adjustments for any changes in the patient's condition or lifestyle.

It is important to educate patients about the various factors that can affect the absorption of Levothyroxine. It is generally advised to take levothyroxine on an empty stomach, preferably 30 to 60 minutes before breakfast. Timing is crucial to ensure maximum absorption, as certain foods and medications may hinder its effectiveness. For example, if you take calcium and iron supplements, soy products, or high-fiber foods at the same time as levothyroxine, it can interfere with its absorption. It is commonly recommended for patients to establish a regular routine, ensuring that they take their medication at a consistent time every day in order to maintain stable hormone levels.

In addition to considering dosage and absorption, it's important to take into account the patient's lifestyle and other medications when assessing the effectiveness of levothyroxine. Healthcare providers need to take into account the possible interactions between levothyroxine and any other medications the patient is currently using. For example, specific antacids, cholesterol-lowering medications, and antidepressants may impact the absorption or metabolism of levothyroxine. Open communication between the patient and their healthcare provider is essential to ensure that any new medications or changes in diet are discussed and managed appropriately.

For many patients, levothyroxine holds the key to regaining their health and vitality. Many people experience noticeable enhancements in their energy levels, mental clarity, and overall well-being when their thyroid hormone levels are balanced. Experiencing relief from the debilitating symptoms of hypothyroidism, such as fatigue, weight gain, and depression, can have a profound impact on individuals' lives. It enables them to resume their daily activities and enjoy a higher quality of life.

Nevertheless, the path with levothyroxine can be quite complex at times. Certain individuals may encounter side effects, especially in the early stages of treatment. These symptoms can include palpitations, an elevated heart rate, feelings of anxiety, and difficulty sleeping, which are often signs of a dosage that may be too high. These symptoms require immediate contact with your healthcare provider, who can make adjustments to the dosage to alleviate these effects. The objective is to discover the ideal dosage that relieves symptoms without producing any negative side effects.

For patients who do not achieve optimal results with levothy-roxine alone, other options to consider include alternative thyroid hormone preparations or combination therapies. These alternatives need to be closely monitored and the dosage needs to be tailored to each individual, as they can make managing thyroid hormone levels more complicated.

Liothyronine (T3) Therapy

Cytomel, also known as liothyronine, is a synthetic version of T3, the active hormone produced by the thyroid gland. Unlike levothyroxine (T4), which requires conversion into T3 within the body, liothyronine provides a direct source of the active hormone without the need for this conversion step. For certain patients, especially those who do not experience complete improvement with T4 therapy alone, liothyronine can make a significant difference, providing better symptom relief and a higher quality of life.

The appeal of liothyronine stems from its strong effectiveness and quick response time. As an expert in the field of endocrinology, it is well known that T3 is the hormone that has the most profound impact on the body. It directly interacts with cells to effectively regulate metabolism, energy production, and a range of bodily functions. If T4 to T3 conversion is hindered, it can result from a range of factors such as genetic variations, chronic illness, or certain medications. In such cases, patients may not fully reap the advantages of levothyroxine. Supplementing with liothyronine can be beneficial in these situations, as it can help achieve optimal thyroid hormone levels and alleviate persistent symptoms.

Commencing liothyronine therapy necessitates thoughtful deliberation and the guidance of a knowledgeable professional. Dosing liothyronine can be more challenging compared to levothyroxine because of its potent and fast-acting properties. It has a shorter half-life, so it doesn't remain in the bloodstream as long as T4. To maintain stable hormone levels, multiple doses throughout the day are usually necessary. Typically, the initial dosage is kept at a low level, usually around 5 micrograms, and then adjusted gradually according to the patient's reaction and laboratory findings.

Individuals undergoing liothyronine therapy frequently experience significant enhancements in their energy levels, mental clarity, and overall sense of well-being. The swift action of T3 can offer a much-needed boost for individuals dealing with persistent fatigue, depression, and cognitive fog, even when

TSH and T4 levels are optimal. Understanding the direct impact of T3 on metabolic processes can be beneficial in addressing weight management, which is often a concern for individuals with hypothyroidism.

Nevertheless, the strength of liothyronine can lead to more noticeable side effects if not properly controlled. Experiencing symptoms like palpitations, anxiety, irritability, and insomnia may occur, particularly when the dosage is excessive. This requires a careful approach to dosing and monitoring, with regular adjustments to achieve the optimal balance. It is crucial to provide patients with information regarding the possible side effects and the significance of following their prescribed dosing schedule.

Combination therapy is a potential role of liothyronine therapy that sets it apart. Certain patients may find it advantageous to use a combination of T4 and T3 hormones. This involves taking levothyroxine to maintain a consistent level of T4 and liothyronine to provide additional active T3. This approach can be especially advantageous for patients who have genetic variations in deiodinase enzymes, which help convert T4 to T3. Combination therapy necessitates precise adjustment and diligent observation to prevent hormone level fluctuations and guarantee effective symptom management.

Although liothyronine is not typically the initial choice for treating hypothyroidism, it can be a beneficial option for patients who don't experience optimal results with levothy-roxine alone. When considering the use of liothyronine, it is important to tailor the decision to each patient's specific needs, considering their individual physiology, symptoms, and previous treatment outcomes. Staying up-to-date with the latest research and clinical guidelines is essential for healthcare providers to effectively incorporate liothyronine into their therapeutic arsenal.

Desiccated Thyroid Extracts

Desiccated thyroid extracts (DTE), commonly referred to as Armour Thyroid or Nature-Throid, offer a more conventional method of addressing hypothyroidism. Unlike synthetic hormone replacements such as levothyroxine, DTE is derived from the dried thyroid glands of pigs. This natural formulation includes a blend of thyroxine (T4), triiodothyronine (T3), and other thyroid hormones, offering a comprehensive hormonal profile that some patients may find to be more effective.

Desiccated thyroid extracts have been used for over a century, making them one of the oldest treatments for hypothyroidism. Prior to the development of synthetic hormones, desiccated thyroid was the main treatment option that existed. With its extensive medical usage over the years, this product has gained a devoted group of patients who value its organic source and wide range of hormones.

Desiccated thyroid extracts offer a significant advantage by containing both T4 and T3 hormones. Unlike synthetic levothyroxine, which only targets T4 and requires conversion to T3 by the body, DTE provides a direct supply of the more potent T3 hormone. This can be especially helpful for patients who struggle with converting T4 to T3, which can be affected by a range of genetic, nutritional, or health-related factors.

Many patients find that desiccated thyroid extracts provide significant relief from symptoms, especially if they do not experience optimal well-being with levothyroxine alone. Having T3 in DTE can result in rapid enhancements in energy levels, cognitive function, and overall vitality. Patients often report feeling a greater sense of well-being and improved overall health when using DTE instead of synthetic alternatives.

Nevertheless, there is ongoing debate surrounding the use of desiccated thyroid extracts. Ensuring consistent potency is a significant challenge when it comes to DTE. Due to its natural origin from animal glands, the hormone levels may differ from batch to batch. Ensuring consistent and accurate hormone content is crucial due to the variability that exists. Some healthcare providers and patients may find this variability concerning, preferring the reliability of synthetic hormones.

In addition, the dosing of DTE may present more complexity compared to synthetic alternatives. The amount of T4 and T3 in each grain of desiccated thyroid extract can vary between brands, with a typical weight of approximately 60-65 mg. It is important to carefully adjust and closely monitor the dosage to determine the most effective amount for each individual. Healthcare providers need a deep understanding of DTE dosing to effectively manage it.

Despite these challenges, numerous patients discover desiccated thyroid extracts to be a highly effective and preferred treatment option. When considering the use of DTE, patients and healthcare providers often engage in a collaborative discussion. They carefully evaluate the advantages of a natural, comprehensive hormone profile while also considering the potential for variability and the importance of precise dosing.

It is essential to educate patients who are considering or using desiccated thyroid extracts. Recognizing the significance of maintaining a consistent medication routine, being aware of possible side effects, and understanding when to seek medical guidance are all vital aspects of successful treatment. It is important for patients to establish a consistent daily routine for taking their medication and to be mindful of certain foods or supplements that may hinder its absorption, like calcium or iron.

Medication Management

Proper management of medication is essential in order to maintain the ideal levels of thyroid hormones and ensure the successful treatment of hypothyroidism. It is important to follow the prescribed medications, regularly monitor your health, and address any factors that could impact the effectiveness of your medication.

Adherence to Medication

Consistently taking prescribed medication is essential for effectively managing hypothyroidism. It is crucial to inform patients about the significance of consistently and regularly taking their thyroid hormone replacement therapy at the same time every day. Consistency in taking medication helps maintain stable hormone levels and prevent the return of symptoms. By incorporating reminders, pill organizers, and a consistent daily routine, adherence can be significantly improved.

Interactions with other medications

Various medications have the potential to interfere with thyroid hormone replacement therapy, which can impact how well it is absorbed and how effective it is. Certain medications and supplements can affect how levothyroxine is absorbed by the body. These include calcium and iron supplements, antacids with aluminum or magnesium, and specific cholesterol-lowering drugs. Patients should always disclose all medications and supplements they are taking to their healthcare provider to prevent any potential interactions. Sometimes, modifying the timing of medication administration can help alleviate these interactions.

Monitoring Thyroid Function

It is crucial to regularly monitor thyroid function to ensure optimal medication management. Regular monitoring of TSH and free T4 levels is important to maintain thyroid hormone levels within the desired range. It is recommended that patients undergo regular thyroid function testing, typically every 6 to 12 months. However, if there are any changes in symptoms, medication, or health status, more frequent testing may be necessary. During pregnancy, it is important to closely monitor pregnant women with hypothyroidism, as their thyroid hormone requirements may increase.

3.2. Alternative Treatments

Although thyroid hormone replacement therapy is a commonly used and effective treatment for hypothyroidism, some patients are interested in exploring complementary and alternative approaches to supplement their treatment. Alternative treatments can provide extra support, particularly for individuals who still have symptoms despite receiving standard medical care.

Herbal and Natural Remedies

Traditional remedies have been relied upon for generations to promote healthy thyroid function and provide relief from hypothyroidism symptoms. Although the effectiveness of these natural approaches may vary according to scientific evidence, numerous patients have reported finding them beneficial when used alongside conventional treatments. It is important to seek guidance from a healthcare professional prior to initiating any herbal or natural remedy, in order to ensure safety and compatibility with prescribed medications.

Ashwagandha

Ashwagandha, scientifically known as Withania somnifera, is a herb highly regarded in Ayurvedic medicine for its wide range of health benefits. This adaptogenic herb has a long history of use, spanning over 3,000 years, for its energy-enhancing, stress-reducing, and vitality-improving properties. In recent times, there has been a growing interest in the West regarding its ability to aid thyroid function, especially in individuals with hypothyroidism.

The effects of Ashwagandha on thyroid health are diverse. It is thought to aid in balancing thyroid hormone levels by providing support to the adrenal glands and reducing long-term stress, both of which play a crucial role in maintaining thyroid health.

According to research, ashwagandha has been found to have a positive impact on thyroid hormone levels. A study was published in the *Journal of Alternative and Complementary Medicine* that examined the impact of ashwagandha root extract on individuals with subclinical hypothyroidism. The study revealed that individuals who took ashwagandha experienced notable enhancements in their T3 and T4 levels in comparison to those who were given a placebo. It suggests that ashwagandha may potentially improve thyroid function and help maintain hormone balance.

Adaptogenic Properties

Ashwagandha falls under the category of adaptogens, aiding the body in adapting to stress and promoting balance. Chronic stress has been found to contribute to thyroid dysfunction by causing imbalances in cortisol and other stress hormones. These imbalances can disrupt the production of thyroid hormones. Reducing stress can have a positive impact on thyroid health, as ashwagandha has been found to support this connection. With its adaptogenic properties, it can effectively regulate the body's stress response, resulting in lower cortisol levels and enhanced overall endocrine function.

Assisting the adrenal glands

The connection between the adrenal glands and thyroid function has been extensively studied and documented. When the adrenal glands are under constant strain from chronic stress, they start to generate an abundance of cortisol, which can have a negative impact on thyroid function. Using Ashwagandha can be beneficial for adrenal health as it helps to lower cortisol levels and enhance the body's ability to handle stress. With its ability to support the adrenal glands, it can help relieve the strain on the thyroid, leading to improved hormone balance.

Ways to Include Ashwagandha in Your Routine

Adding ashwagandha to your daily routine can be easy and advantageous. It is offered in different forms such as capsules, powders, and liquid extracts, providing a range of options to fit your lifestyle.

Ashwagandha capsules offer convenience and a consistent intake with their standardized dose. Adding powders to smoothies, teas, or other beverages provides a versatile alternative for individuals who would rather not consume pills. Liquid extracts are an alternative that the body can absorb more rapidly.

Determining the suitable dosage of ashwagandha can differ based on individual requirements and health circumstances. Studies indicate that a daily dose of 300–600 mg of ashwagandha extract may be beneficial for enhancing thyroid function and alleviating stress. Starting with a lower dose and gradually increasing it, while keeping a close eye on your body's response and any possible side effects, is vital.

Ashwagandha can be used alongside conventional thyroid treatments, such as levothyroxine. It is important to seek guidance from a healthcare professional before incorporating ashwagandha into your routine, particularly if you are taking thyroid medication. Your healthcare provider can assist in determining the correct dosage and closely monitor your thyroid hormone levels to ensure the most effective treatment.

Although ashwagandha is generally safe for most individuals, it is important to be aware of certain precautions. It is advised against pregnant or breastfeeding women due to a lack of safety data. Furthermore, it is important for those with autoimmune thyroid conditions, like Hashimoto's thyroiditis, to exercise caution when using ashwagandha, as it has the potential to stimulate the immune system.

Occasionally, ashwagandha may cause gastrointestinal discomfort, diarrhea, or trigger allergic reactions, although these side effects are uncommon. If you encounter any negative reactions, it is crucial to stop using the product and seek guidance from a medical professional.

The Science Behind Ashwagandha

There has been a significant increase in scientific interest in ashwagandha in recent years, with a multitude of studies investigating its potential health benefits. The active compounds in ashwagandha, called withanolides, are thought to be the cause of its therapeutic effects. These compounds have demonstrated anti-inflammatory, antioxidant, and neuroprotective properties, which can enhance overall health and well-being.

A study in the Journal of Ethnopharmacology showcased the potential of ashwagandha to improve thyroid function in animal models. Researchers noted a rise in serum T4 concentrations, indicating that ashwagandha may have a stimulating effect on the thyroid gland. Further research is necessary to validate these effects in humans, but the results are encouraging.

A study published in the Indian Journal of Psychological Medicine investigated the impact of ashwagandha on stress and anxiety. The study revealed noteworthy decreases in cortisol levels and enhancements in stress and anxiety symptoms among participants who received ashwagandha, in comparison to those in the placebo group. These stress-reducing effects can indirectly support thyroid health by mitigating the effects of chronic stress on the endocrine system.

For optimal thyroid health, it is important to incorporate Ashwagandha into a comprehensive approach to overall well-being. It is important to maintain a well-rounded lifestyle, which involves a healthy diet, consistent physical activity, effective stress management, and sufficient rest. Through understanding the underlying factors behind thyroid dysfunction and prioritizing overall well-being, individuals can experience enhanced results and a higher standard of living.

Selenium

Selenium is an essential trace mineral that is vital for maintaining optimal thyroid function. Despite being needed in small quantities, its effect on thyroid health is significant. Selenium plays a crucial role in the thyroid by being a key component of selenoproteins. These enzymes are vital for the production and regulation of thyroid hormones. Understanding the intricacies of selenium's role and its benefits allows us to recognize the importance of this mineral for individuals dealing with hypothyroidism.

Selenium supports the functioning of certain enzymes called selenoproteins, such as glutathione peroxidases and iodothyronine deiodinases. These enzymes have multiple functions:

Conversion of Thyroid Hormones

Selenium helps convert thyroxine (T4) into the more potent triiodothyronine (T3). This conversion is facilitated by the enzyme iodothyronine deiodinase, which relies on selenium. If selenium levels are insufficient, the body might have difficulty in producing enough T3, which could worsen symptoms of hypothyroidism.

Antioxidant Protection

Understanding the importance of incorporating selenium into glutathione peroxidases is essential for safeguarding the thyroid gland against oxidative damage. It is worth noting that the thyroid gland generates hydrogen peroxide during the process of synthesizing thyroid hormones. Enzymes that rely on selenium have a key role in neutralizing this potentially harmful substance, safeguarding the gland and promoting optimal hormone production.

Immune System Regulation

Selenium also has an impact on regulating the immune system. It enhances the body's capacity to address autoimmune conditions, including Hashimoto's thyroiditis, a primary contributor to hypothyroidism. Having sufficient selenium levels can be beneficial in managing inflammation and potentially decreasing the autoimmune response targeting the thyroid gland.

Foods that Contain Selenium

It is important to maintain a proper selenium intake in order to promote optimal thyroid function. Obtaining selenium from food sources is generally preferred due to its bioavailability and added nutritional benefits, rather than relying on supplements.

Brazil nuts are a delicious and nutritious snack that can provide numerous health benefits. They are packed with essential nutrients like selenium, magnesium, and vitamin E. Incorporating Brazil nuts into your diet can support heart health, boost immunity, and promote healthy skin. They are known for their high selenium content, making them a valuable addition to your diet. Just a few Brazil nuts can easily provide more than the recommended daily intake of selenium, making them a convenient and effective way to increase selenium levels.

Seafood and fish

Fish and seafood are great choices for obtaining selenium. These types of fish, such as tuna, halibut, sardines, and shrimp, are known for their rich content of this important mineral. Adding these to your diet can help you maintain optimal selenium levels and support thyroid function.

Meat and poultry

Organ meats, like liver, along with muscle meats such as beef, chicken, and turkey, are excellent sources of selenium. These foods offer a range of vital nutrients that contribute to overall well-being.

Selenium Supplementation

If individuals struggle to get sufficient selenium from their diet alone, supplementation can be a helpful solution. It is important to exercise caution when considering selenium supplementation, as high doses can lead to potential toxicity.

The daily recommended amount of selenium for adults is approximately 55 micrograms. Supplements usually have dosages that range from 50 to 200 micrograms. It is crucial to follow the suggested dosage and seek guidance from a healthcare professional prior to beginning supplementation to prevent the possibility of selenium toxicity.

Excessive intake of selenium can lead to toxicity, although this is quite rare. Common signs of selenium toxicity may manifest as gastrointestinal discomfort, hair loss, the appearance of white blotchy nails, and a distinct odor resembling garlic on the breath. Regular monitoring of selenium levels through blood tests can help ensure the safety and effectiveness of supplementation.

Scientific evidence that supports the benefits of selenium

Multiple studies highlight the advantages of selenium for maintaining thyroid health. As an expert in the field of endocrinology, I would like to highlight a study published in the Journal of Clinical Endocrinology & Metabolism. This research discovered that selenium supplementation had a significant impact on reducing thyroid peroxidase antibodies (TPOAb) in individuals with Hashimoto's thyroiditis. Lower TPOAb levels indicate a decrease in autoimmune activity targeting the thyroid gland.

A recent study published in the European Journal of Endocrinology emphasized the significance of selenium in safeguarding against goiter and thyroid dysfunction in populations with low selenium levels. Research indicates that selenium supplementation may be beneficial for maintaining thyroid health, especially in regions with limited dietary selenium intake.

Practical Steps for Implementing Selenium

Adding selenium to your daily routine can be easy and advantageous. Here are some practical steps you can take to ensure you're getting enough selenium:

1. Balanced Diet: Emphasize the importance of maintaining a well-rounded diet that incorporates foods high in selenium. It is important to include a range of sources in your diet, such as nuts, seafood, and meats, to ensure you are getting a wide variety of nutrients.
2. Regular Monitoring: Collaborate with your healthcare provider to keep a close eye on your selenium levels, particularly if you are thinking about taking supplements.

Regular blood tests can assist in customizing your intake to meet your individual requirements while staying within safe limits.

3. Lifestyle Integration: Implement gradual, long-lasting adjustments to your diet and lifestyle. For example, it's a good idea to have a jar of Brazil nuts within reach for a convenient and healthy snack. Another option is to incorporate selenium-rich fish or poultry into your meal planning.

If you decide to go for supplements, it's important to select high-quality products from well-known brands. Follow the suggested dosages and consult with your healthcare provider to safely incorporate supplementation into your routine.

Iodine

Iodine is a trace element that plays a vital role in maintaining thyroid health. This mineral supports the production of thyroid hormones, which are responsible for regulating various bodily functions such as metabolism, growth, and development. Despite its significance, iodine deficiency continues to be a major global health concern, impacting millions of individuals, especially in regions with iodine-deficient soil. Now, we will explore the crucial role of iodine in maintaining proper thyroid function, including its sources, the consequences of a deficiency, and practical measures to ensure sufficient intake.

The Importance of Iodine in Thyroid Function

Iodine is essential for the production of thyroid hormones thyroxine (T4) and triiodothyronine (T3). The thyroid gland absorbs iodine from the bloodstream and incorporates it into these hormones. Around 80% of the iodine in our body is stored in the thyroid gland, highlighting its crucial importance in maintaining thyroid health.

The process starts with the absorption of iodine by the thyroid gland, which is later used to create T4 and T3 by combining with the amino acid tyrosine. The thyroid gland primarily produces T4, which consists of four iodine atoms. It is then transformed into T3, which is the more active form, within the body's tissues.

Thyroid hormones, fueled by iodine, play a crucial role in the control of metabolism. They help enhance the rate at which cells convert nutrients into energy, thereby impacting basal metabolic rate (BMR). This regulation has a significant influence on energy levels, weight management, and temperature control, highlighting the wide-ranging impact of iodine on overall health.

Where to Find Iodine

Although iodine deficiency is less prevalent in developed countries because of iodized salt, it can still occur, especially in people with specific dietary restrictions or those residing in regions with low iodine levels.

The introduction of iodized salt has been a remarkable achievement in public health, leading to a significant decrease in the occurrence of iodine deficiency disorders (IDD) on a global scale. Including iodine in table salt offers a straightforward and efficient method to guarantee sufficient iodine consumption. Incorporating a daily intake of iodized salt can effectively fulfill the body's iodine needs.

Seafood is a great choice for those looking to boost their iodine intake through their diet. Fish like cod, tuna, and shrimp have a notably high iodine content. Seaweed, like various types such as kelp, nori, and wakame, is highly abundant in iodine, often exceeding the recommended daily intake in just one serving.

Dairy products like milk, cheese, and yogurt are known to be rich in iodine. This is because dairy cows are often given iodine supplements and iodine-containing disinfectants are used during dairy processing.

Eggs, especially the yolks, are a good source of iodine. Adding eggs to your diet can help boost your iodine intake.

Some grains and vegetables, particularly those cultivated in soil with high iodine content, can offer a moderate supply of iodine. Nevertheless, the amount of iodine found in these foods can differ significantly based on the iodine levels in the soil where they are cultivated.

The Effects of Iodine Deficiency

Insufficient iodine levels can result in a range of health problems, specifically impacting the thyroid gland. Goiter, an enlargement of the thyroid gland, is a widely recognized condition caused by iodine deficiency. Nevertheless, the consequences of insufficient iodine go beyond goiter and can lead to a range of metabolic and developmental disorders.

Goiter

When the thyroid gland enlarges, it is because it is trying to capture more iodine from the bloodstream in order to produce enough thyroid hormones. Although goiters are typically not painful, they may lead to discomfort, difficulties with swallowing, and breathing problems if they grow in size.

Hypothyroidism

Severe iodine deficiency can result in hypothyroidism, which is marked by inadequate production of thyroid hormones. Common symptoms may include feelings of tiredness, unexplained weight gain, sensitivity to cold temperatures, and difficulties with cognitive function. If iodine deficiency is not addressed and hypothyroidism is left untreated, it can result in more serious health complications.

Cretinism

Iodine deficiency during pregnancy can have severe consequences for the developing fetus. If iodine deficiency is severe during pregnancy, it can lead to cretinism, a condition characterized by significant delays in mental and physical development. Even a slight lack of iodine can negatively impact the cognitive abilities of children.

Impaired Cognitive Function

Iodine plays a vital role in the development of the brain, especially during the crucial stages of fetal development and early childhood. Insufficient iodine intake may result in cognitive impairments, lower IQ, and delays in development. It is crucial to ensure sufficient iodine intake during pregnancy and childhood to support optimal cognitive development.

Practical Steps to Ensure Sufficient Iodine Intake

It is important to maintain a balanced approach when it comes to ensuring sufficient iodine intake, which includes incorporating dietary sources and, if needed, supplements. Here are some practical steps you can take to ensure your iodine levels stay at a healthy level:

1. Incorporate Iodized Salt: Using iodized salt in cooking and at the table is a straightforward method to guarantee sufficient iodine intake. It is important to maintain a proper balance between iodine and sodium intake, as consuming too much salt can result in various health problems like hypertension.
2. Enjoy Seafood: Adding seafood to your diet a few times a week can greatly increase your iodine intake. Fish, shellfish, and seaweed are fantastic sources of iodine and offer extra nutritional benefits, including omega-3 fatty acids.

3. Include dairy products and eggs: Consuming dairy products on a regular basis can help boost your iodine levels. Include a range of dairy products, like milk, cheese, and yogurt, in your diet for optimal nutrition. Eggs are a versatile and nutritious food that can contribute to meeting your iodine requirements. Indulge in the delightful versatility of eggs, whether they're boiled, scrambled, or incorporated into your beloved recipes.

Bladderwrack

Bladderwrack, also known as Fucus vesiculosus, is a remarkable brown seaweed that has been highly regarded throughout history due to its numerous medicinal properties. Bladderwrack, discovered in coastal areas such as the North Sea, western Baltic Sea, and the Atlantic and Pacific Oceans, has garnered attention in the contemporary health community due to its potential advantages in promoting thyroid health. This marine algae is known for its high iodine content, which is important for maintaining healthy thyroid function.

Bladderwrack is packed with a wide range of nutrients, including iodine, as well as an array of other minerals, vitamins, and beneficial compounds. This seaweed is a fantastic source of:

1. **Iodine:** Consuming bladderwrack can be beneficial for

maintaining proper iodine levels, which in turn supports healthy thyroid function.

2. **Fucoidan:** Fucoidan is a polysaccharide that is commonly found in brown seaweeds such as bladderwrack. This substance has been extensively researched for its potential to reduce inflammation, combat viruses, and enhance the immune system. These benefits can enhance overall health and well-being, bolstering the body's capacity to handle stress and illness.

3. **Alginate:** Alginate, a compound present in bladderwrack, has the remarkable ability to effectively bind heavy metals and other toxins, thereby assisting in the process of detoxification. Implementing these strategies can have a positive impact on the body's toxic load, leading to improved thyroid function and overall health.

The Importance of Bladderwrack in Maintaining Thyroid Health

Bladderwrack is highly beneficial for promoting thyroid health, especially in individuals with hypothyroidism or iodine deficiency. Bladderwrack has several potential benefits for thyroid function:

Enhancing Iodine Levels

For those who have low iodine levels, adding bladderwrack to your diet can be beneficial in increasing iodine levels. This can help ensure that the thyroid gland has enough raw materials to produce sufficient thyroid hormones. These methods can provide relief from symptoms commonly associated with hypothyroidism, including fatigue, weight gain, and cold intolerance.

Supporting Hormone Balance

Bladderwrack's iodine content is beneficial for maintaining a balanced production of T4 and T3 hormones, which helps support overall hormonal equilibrium. Having a proper balance is important for maintaining metabolic regulation, energy levels, and overall well-being.

Anti-inflammatory Properties

Bladderwrack contains anti-inflammatory compounds, including fucoidan, which can effectively reduce inflammation in the thyroid gland. This is especially advantageous for individuals who have autoimmune thyroid conditions, such as Hashimoto's thyroiditis. Bladderwrack has the potential to reduce inflammation and provide support for improved thyroid function by addressing the autoimmune attack on the thyroid.

Support for Detoxification

Alginate's capacity to effectively bind to heavy metals and toxins is beneficial for facilitating the detoxification process. Minimizing the body's exposure to harmful substances can promote optimal thyroid function, as these toxins have the potential to disrupt the production and effectiveness of thyroid hormones.

Ways to Include Bladderwrack in Your Routine

Bladderwrack can be easily included in different forms in your diet, providing a natural way to enhance your thyroid health.

It can be found in various supplement forms, such as capsules and powders. These supplements offer a convenient method to include bladderwrack in your everyday regimen. When it comes to selecting supplements, it's important to opt for high-quality products from well-known brands to guarantee their purity and potency.

Bladderwrack tea is a commonly chosen method for consuming this seaweed. You can make the tea by steeping dried bladderwrack in hot water. Regularly consuming bladderwrack tea can help increase iodine levels and offer various health benefits linked to this seaweed.

Bladderwrack can also be incorporated into culinary preparations, much like other types of seaweed. It can be incorporated into soups, stews, and salads, offering a distinctive taste and a nutritional boost. Adding bladderwrack to your meals can help you maintain a consistent supply of iodine and other beneficial compounds.

Safety and Precautions

It is important to exercise caution when using bladderwrack due to its potential impact on iodine intake, despite its many health benefits. Consuming too much iodine can result in thyroid dysfunction, which may include hyperthyroidism and thyroiditis. It is important to seek guidance from a healthcare professional prior to beginning bladderwrack, especially if you have preexisting thyroid conditions or are currently taking thyroid medications.

Possible Adverse Reactions

Bladderwrack is typically considered safe for most individuals when consumed in moderate quantities. Nevertheless, there may be some adverse effects such as gastrointestinal discomfort, allergic reactions, and thyroid dysfunction if consumed excessively. By closely monitoring your intake and seeking guidance from a healthcare professional, you can effectively reduce these risks.

Medication Interactions

Bladderwrack can potentially have interactions with specific medications, such as thyroid hormone replacements and anticoagulants. If you are currently on any medications, it is essential to have a conversation with your healthcare provider regarding the use of bladderwrack to prevent any potential adverse interactions.

Scientific Research on Bladderwrack

There has been a significant increase in scientific interest surrounding bladderwrack, as researchers have been investigating its potential advantages for thyroid health and other areas. A study published in the Journal of Medicinal Food emphasized the antioxidant and anti-inflammatory properties of bladderwrack, suggesting its potential in addressing oxidative stress and inflammation.

A study published in the Journal of Ethnopharmacology investigated the iodine levels in different types of seaweeds, including bladderwrack. The study found that bladderwrack has a high concentration of iodine, which further supports its potential as a natural iodine supplement. These studies offer a scientific foundation for the traditional use of bladderwrack in promoting thyroid health.

Guggul

Guggul, obtained from the resin of the Mukul myrrh tree (Commiphora mukul), has been widely used in Ayurvedic medicine for centuries. Guggul is becoming increasingly recognized for its potential benefits in supporting thyroid health, especially in managing hypothyroidism. It is well-known for its potent anti-inflammatory and cholesterol-lowering properties. This ancient remedy has a one-of-a-kind composition and a range of effects that make it an intriguing natural choice for individuals looking to improve their thyroid function and overall well-being.

Guggul contains guggulsterones, which are plant steroids that have been extensively researched for their therapeutic properties. These compounds are thought to influence the activity of nuclear hormone receptors, which are key in controlling metabolism, inflammation, and hormone balance.

Boosting Thyroid Activity

Guggul has a fascinating ability to enhance thyroid function. Studies have indicated that guggulsterones have the potential to boost the functioning of the thyroid gland, leading to an increase in the production of thyroid hormones. Guggul is especially beneficial for individuals with hypothyroidism, as it helps to increase thyroid hormone levels. By increasing the production of these hormones, guggul can assist in relieving common symptoms of hypothyroidism like fatigue, weight gain, and mental fog.

Managing Cholesterol Levels

Guggul is well-known for its cholesterol-regulating properties, in addition to its effects on thyroid stimulation. Hypothyroidism frequently results in increased levels of low-density lipoprotein (LDL) cholesterol, which is commonly known as "bad" cholesterol. Research has demonstrated the ability of guggulsterones to improve the breakdown of LDL cholesterol in the liver, facilitating its removal from the bloodstream. With its ability to support thyroid function and lower cholesterol, guggul is a natural remedy that can greatly improve cardiovascular health for those with hypothyroidism.

Purification and Detoxification

Many practitioners of Ayurveda frequently utilize guggul due to its detoxifying properties. Many people believe that it has the ability to cleanse the blood, eliminate toxins, and enhance overall well-being. This cleansing action can be especially advantageous for maintaining optimal thyroid health by reducing the accumulation of harmful toxins that may disrupt thyroid function.

Anti-inflammatory and Analgesic Effects

The anti-inflammatory and analgesic properties of Guggul have been extensively documented. Inflammation is a frequent concern in thyroid disorders, especially in autoimmune conditions such as Hashimoto's thyroiditis. Guggul has the potential to reduce inflammation and enhance the function of the thyroid gland. The analgesic effects of this treatment can help alleviate the joint and muscle pain commonly experienced with hypothyroidism.

Recent Studies on Guggul

Scientific research in recent times has started to confirm the traditional uses of guggul, specifically its positive effects on thyroid health and lipid metabolism. A study in the Journal of Ethnopharmacology revealed that guggulsterones have the potential to boost thyroid function and improve the conversion of T4 to T3, which is the active form of thyroid hormone. This discovery provides further evidence for the effectiveness of guggul as a natural treatment for hypothyroidism.

A recent study published in the Journal of Cardiovascular Pharmacology emphasized the lipid-lowering effects of guggul. Studies have shown that guggulsterones have the potential to lower LDL cholesterol levels and enhance the lipid profile, which plays a vital role in managing the cardiovascular risks linked to hypothyroidism.

Ways to Include Guggul in Your Routine

Incorporating guggul into your health routine can be achieved through different options, such as capsules, powders, and traditional Ayurvedic preparations.

Guggul supplements are easily found in the market, often with standardized levels of guggulsterones. These supplements offer a convenient and accurate method of consuming guggul. It is important to adhere to the dosage instructions on the product label and seek guidance from a healthcare provider to determine the suitable dose for your requirements.

Ayurvedic Formulations

Guggul is a crucial component in numerous traditional Ayurvedic preparations. One formulation that can be considered is "Kaishore Guggul," which is known for its detoxifying properties and its ability to promote joint health. One option is "Kanchanar Guggul," a specialized formulation designed to promote healthy thyroid function and address imbalances in the glands. These formulations can be taken as directed by a knowledgeable practitioner, who can customize the treatment to your specific condition.

Guggul Powder

You can mix guggul powder with water, honey, or ghee and consume it directly. This conventional approach offers the convenience of adaptable dosing and seamless integration into everyday schedules. Combining guggul with a sweetener like honey can help to mask its pungent and bitter taste, making it more enjoyable to consume.

Safety and Precautions

Although guggul is generally safe for most individuals, it is important to exercise caution when using it, especially if you are taking other medications or have pre-existing health conditions.

It is worth noting that guggul may cause gastrointestinal discomfort, including symptoms like nausea or diarrhea. In some instances, allergic reactions may occur, such as skin rash or itching. If you encounter any negative reactions, it is crucial to stop using it and seek advice from a healthcare professional.

Medication Interactions

It's important to be aware that Guggul can have interactions with specific medications, such as anticoagulants, antiplatelet drugs, and thyroid medications. Informing your healthcare provider about all the supplements and medications you are taking is essential to prevent any potential interactions.

It is advised to avoid using Guggul during pregnancy and breastfeeding as there is insufficient safety data available. It is advisable for women who are pregnant or nursing to consult with their healthcare provider before using guggul.

Conclusion

As we conclude our exploration of treatment options for hypothyroidism, it becomes evident that a comprehensive approach is essential for effectively managing this condition. Conventional treatments, such as thyroid hormone replacement therapy with levothyroxine, form the backbone of hypothyroidism management, providing a reliable and consistent means to restore normal thyroid function. Personalized dosing and regular monitoring are crucial components of this conventional approach, ensuring that treatment is tailored to meet the unique needs of each individual.

However, the journey to optimal thyroid health often extends beyond conventional medicine. Alternative treatments, including herbal remedies like ashwagandha, selenium, iodine, bladderwrack, and guggul, offer additional support and can enhance the overall effectiveness of thyroid management. These natural remedies, rooted in ancient traditions and supported by modern research, provide valuable options for those seeking a holistic approach to their health.

Ultimately, the most effective approach to managing hypothyroidism is one that combines the strengths of conventional medicine with the benefits of alternative therapies and lifestyle modifications. By adopting a holistic and individualized treatment plan, patients can navigate their journey toward optimal thyroid health with greater confidence and success. This comprehensive strategy not only addresses the symptoms of hypothyroidism but also promotes overall health and well-being, empowering individuals to lead healthier, more fulfilling lives.

4

Diet and Nutrition

"You are what you eat." This adage holds particularly true when it comes to managing thyroid health. For those living with hypothyroidism, understanding the connection between diet and thyroid function is essential. According to the American Thyroid Association, millions of people worldwide suffer from thyroid disorders, with hypothyroidism being the most common. Proper nutrition can significantly impact the effectiveness of treatment, symptom management, and overall quality of life.

In this chapter, we explore the importance of diet in thyroid health, focusing on the essential nutrients that support thyroid function and the foods that can enhance or hinder this process. From the significance of iodine and selenium—detailed in earlier sections—to the roles of zinc, iron, vitamin D, omega-3 fatty acids, and B vitamins, we delve into how these nutrients contribute to a healthy thyroid. We also address foods to avoid or consume in moderation, such as goitrogenic foods, gluten, processed foods, and excessive caffeine and alcohol, to prevent interference with thyroid function.

Additionally, we provide comprehensive dietary plans and practical recipes tailored to support thyroid health. These meal plans are designed to ensure balanced nutrient intake, optimize thyroid function, and promote overall well-being. By understanding the impact of diet on thyroid health and implementing these practical strategies, individuals with hypothyroidism can take proactive steps to manage their condition and improve their quality of life.

4.1. Importance of Diet in Thyroid Health

The connection between diet and thyroid health is extremely important. For individuals with thyroid disorders, especially hypothyroidism, diet plays a crucial role in managing the condition and maximizing thyroid function. This section explores the importance of diet in maintaining thyroid health, discussing the necessary nutrients for optimal thyroid function, as well as recommending specific foods to incorporate and avoid. It also offers practical advice to improve overall well-being.

We already talked about two essential nutrients, iodine, and selenium (see subchapter 3.2.), so we'll not discuss them in this section.

Nutrients Essential for Thyroid Function

Proper nutrition is essential for the thyroid gland to efficiently produce hormones and sustain its optimal function. Gaining knowledge about these essential nutrients and integrating them into one's diet can have a profound effect on the well-being of the thyroid and help alleviate the symptoms associated with hypothyroidism.

Zinc

Zinc plays a crucial role in various cellular metabolic processes, such as the synthesis and regulation of thyroid hormones. This mineral supports the functioning of deiodinase enzymes, responsible for converting thyroxine (T4) into the more potent triiodothyronine (T3). Insufficient zinc can hinder this conversion process, resulting in an imbalance in thyroid hormone levels and worsening symptoms of hypothyroidism.

Zinc is vital for maintaining a strong immune system, especially for those with autoimmune thyroid conditions such as Hashimoto's thyroiditis. Zinc helps regulate the immune response, which can help lower the chances of autoimmune attacks on the thyroid gland. An effectively regulated immune system plays a crucial role in preserving thyroid health and halting the advancement of thyroid disorders.

It is important to maintain a well-rounded diet that includes foods high in zinc to ensure adequate zinc intake. Lean meats such as beef and pork, along with shellfish like oysters and crab, are great sources of zinc. It is worth mentioning that the bioavailability of zinc from plant sources is lower because of the presence of phytates, which can hinder zinc absorption.

Iron

Iron is an essential mineral that plays a crucial role in the production of thyroid hormones, which are vital for thyroid health. Iron supports the process of thyroid peroxidase, an enzyme that facilitates the iodination of tyrosine residues during the synthesis of T4. An iron deficiency can hinder the function of this enzyme, resulting in a decrease in thyroid hormone production and the worsening of symptoms associated with hypothyroidism.

Iron deficiency is a widespread nutritional issue that affects many people, especially women of childbearing age and those with limited access to iron-rich foods. The symptoms of iron deficiency, including fatigue, weakness, and cognitive impairments, can sometimes be similar to those experienced by individuals with hypothyroidism. This can make it even more challenging for people with thyroid disorders to manage their health.

For optimal iron levels, it's essential to incorporate a variety of iron sources into your diet. Animal products such as red meat, poultry, and fish contain heme iron, which is easily absorbed by the body. On the other hand, plant-based foods like lentils, beans, tofu, and spinach contain non-heme iron, which is not as easily absorbed.

Pairing these foods with vitamin C-rich foods, such as citrus fruits, bell peppers, and tomatoes, can enhance the absorption of iron. For instance, incorporating lemon juice or including strawberries can greatly enhance the absorption of iron. On the other hand, it's recommended to steer clear of consuming calcium-rich foods and beverages, like dairy products, along-side iron-rich meals. This is because calcium has the potential to hinder iron absorption.

Vitamin D

Vitamin D, known as the "sunshine vitamin," is essential for maintaining overall health and has specific advantages for thyroid function. This particular vitamin has a special quality – it can be produced by the skin when it is exposed to sunlight.

Vitamin D plays a key role in more than just bone health. It is vital for regulating the immune system, which is especially significant for those with autoimmune thyroid conditions like Hashimoto's thyroiditis.

The immune system modulation of vitamin D is vital for maintaining thyroid health. Studies have indicated a high occurrence of vitamin D deficiency among people with autoim-mune thyroid disorders. Having sufficient levels of vitamin D help maintain a balanced immune response, which can lower the risk of autoimmune attacks on the thyroid gland. This regulation has the potential to alleviate inflammation and safeguard the thyroid tissue, thereby promoting improved thyroid function.

Although sunlight is the most effective way to obtain vitamin D, various factors such as where you live, your skin color and your lifestyle can restrict your sun exposure. This may require you to rely on dietary sources and supplements. Rich sources of vitamin D include fatty fish like salmon, mackerel, and sardines. Fortified foods, such as dairy products, orange juice, and cereals, also play a role in our dietary intake. For those who don't get much sun or have a limited diet, taking vitamin D supplements might be necessary to keep their levels in check. (ideal vitamin D levels are between 50-70 ng/ml)

Omega-3 Fatty Acids

Omega-3 fatty acids have gained considerable recognition for their anti-inflammatory properties and numerous health benefits. These polyunsaturated fats help reduce inflamma-tion, which is often a concern in thyroid disorders, especially autoimmune conditions such as Hashimoto's thyroiditis.

Chronic inflammation can worsen thyroid dysfunction and play a role in the development of autoimmune thyroid diseases. Omega-3 fatty acids, commonly found in fatty fish, have been shown to effectively reduce inflammation by regulating the production of inflammatory cytokines. Reducing inflammation can help alleviate symptoms and promote healthier thyroid function.

People with hypothyroidism commonly experience a higher likelihood of developing cardiovascular problems, such as elevated cholesterol levels and heart disease. Omega-3 fatty acids have been extensively studied for their positive impact on cardiovascular health. They have been found to effectively lower triglyceride levels, reduce blood pressure, and promote overall heart well-being. Omega-3s have an indirect positive impact on individuals with thyroid disorders by promoting cardiovascular health.

Including omega-3-rich foods in your diet is crucial for maximizing their advantages. Fatty fish like salmon, mackerel, and sardines are excellent sources of omega-3s. If fish is not part of your diet, you can incorporate omega-3 supplements like fish oil or algae oil into one's diet can be beneficial in maintaining sufficient intake, especially for those with dietary limitations.

B Vitamins

Water-soluble vitamins known as B vitamins are essential for energy production, metabolism, and maintaining cellular function. For individuals with thyroid disorders, vitamins B12 and B6 play a crucial role in maintaining health.

Vitamin B12 supports the formation of red blood cells, DNA

synthesis, and maintaining proper neurological function. Insufficient levels of B12 can result in anemia, fatigue, and cognitive impairments, which are frequently observed in people with hypothyroidism. Ensuring sufficient intake of B12 can help alleviate these symptoms, enhancing energy levels and cognitive function.

Vitamin B6 plays a crucial role in protein metabolism and the synthesis of neurotransmitters. Additionally, it contributes to the production of thyroid hormones. Having sufficient levels of B6 can help maintain a healthy hormonal balance and support the proper functioning of the thyroid gland.

B vitamins can be found in a wide range of foods. Vitamin B12 is mainly present in animal-derived foods like meat, fish, poultry, eggs, and dairy products. Fortified foods and supplements are crucial for vegetarians and vegans to obtain B12. Vitamin B6 is present in a variety of foods such as poultry, fish, potatoes, and bananas. Including these foods in your diet can help maintain adequate levels of B vitamins and support thyroid health.

Foods to Optimize Thyroid Health

It is essential to include foods that are rich in nutrients in your diet to support thyroid function and maintain good overall health. Here are some dietary recommendations for individuals with hypothyroidism:

Seafood and seaweed

Seafood and seaweed are great options for obtaining iodine. Fish like cod, tuna, and shrimp contain a wealth of iodine and other vital nutrients. Seaweed, such as kelp, nori, and wakame, contains a substantial amount of iodine, which can greatly benefit thyroid health. Adding these foods to your diet can help ensure you get enough iodine, as we covered earlier in this chapter.

Nuts and seeds

Various types of nuts and seeds, such as Brazil nuts, sunflower seeds, and pumpkin seeds, contain significant amounts of selenium and zinc. Consuming a few Brazil nuts daily can meet your recommended daily selenium intake. Including a range of nuts and seeds in your diet can contribute to maintaining healthy thyroid function and supplying important nutrients.

Meats

Beef and poultry, such as chicken and turkey, provide essential nutrients like zinc and iron. These proteins play a crucial role in supporting thyroid hormone synthesis and maintaining optimal metabolic health. Adding lean meats to your diet is essential for getting enough of these important nutrients.

Leafy Greens and Vegetables

Leafy greens and vegetables, such as spinach, kale, and Swiss chard, are packed with vital vitamins and minerals. These foods are beneficial for maintaining thyroid health and promoting overall well-being. Adding a diverse array of vibrant vegetables to your meals guarantees a plethora of essential nutrients and powerful antioxidants.

Grains

Grains like rice, quinoa, and oats, offer a wealth of vital nutrients and fiber. Although they can provide energy, it's crucial to consume them in moderation and opt for gluten-free alternatives if you have a sensitivity or autoimmune thyroid condition.

Fruits and berries

Fruits and berries contain a variety of essential nutrients, including vitamins, antioxidants, and fiber. Berries, especially, contain a significant amount of antioxidants that aid in shielding the thyroid gland against oxidative stress. Adding a range of fruits and berries to your diet can contribute to your overall well-being and supply vital nutrients.

Dairy products

Dairy products, like milk, cheese, and yogurt, provide a rich supply of iodine and vitamin D. They have the ability to provide assistance in maintaining thyroid function and promoting optimal bone health.

Foods to Limit or Remove

It is important to be aware of specific foods that can disrupt thyroid function when managing thyroid health, especially in cases of hypothyroidism. Certain foods can have a negative impact on thyroid health by interfering with hormone production, iodine absorption, or autoimmune responses.

Goitrocenic Foods

Some foods contain naturally occurring substances called goitrogens that can disrupt the normal functioning of the thyroid gland. They can interfere with the absorption of iodine, which is essential for the production of thyroid hormones, potentially causing thyroid problems. Although these foods could be incorporated into a balanced diet, it is important to exercise moderation and employ proper preparation methods to reduce their potential effects.

Cruciferous vegetables

Cruciferous vegetables, like broccoli, cauliflower, Brussels sprouts, cabbage, and kale, are packed with nutrients, but it's worth noting that they also contain goitrogens. These compounds have the potential to disrupt thyroid function by blocking the absorption of iodine. Nevertheless, these vegetables offer a wealth of fiber, vitamins, and antioxidants that contribute to one's overall well-being. When cruciferous vegetables are cooked, their goitrogenic properties are reduced, which is beneficial for people with thyroid issues.

Soy products

Soy products, such as tofu, tempeh, edamame, and soy milk, contain isoflavones that have goitrogenic properties. Research has shown that isoflavones have the potential to disrupt the synthesis of thyroid hormones and hinder the thyroid's ability to absorb iodine. Individuals with hypothyroidism shouldn't consume soy products.

Gluten

Individuals with autoimmune thyroid conditions such as Hashimoto's thyroiditis may experience difficulties with gluten, a protein commonly found in wheat, barley, and rye. There is compelling evidence indicating a connection between gluten sensitivity and autoimmune thyroid disease. Consuming gluten has been found to worsen inflammation and activate immune responses that can negatively impact the thyroid.

For individuals with autoimmune thyroid conditions, following a gluten-free diet has been shown to decrease inflammation and enhance thyroid function. Avoid foods such as bread, pasta, cereals, and baked goods that contain wheat, barley, or rye is recommended to prioritize thyroid health.

Processed Foods

Consuming processed foods, which are frequently packed with

unhealthy fats, sugars, and additives, can have a detrimental effect on thyroid health and overall well-being. These foods have the potential to contribute to weight gain, insulin resistance, and inflammation, which can worsen symptoms associated with hypothyroidism.

Processed foods frequently include significant amounts of refined sugars, leading to abrupt increases in blood sugar and insulin levels. Insulin resistance and weight gain are frequently experienced by individuals with hypothyroidism. Properly managing blood sugar levels is essential for maintaining optimal energy levels and overall metabolic health.

Unhealthy Fats

Consuming trans fats, which are often present in processed and fried foods, can lead to inflammation and interfere with metabolic function. Unhealthy fats can have a detrimental effect on cardiovascular health, which is particularly worrisome for individuals with hypothyroidism who already face a higher risk of heart disease.

Additives and Preservatives

Processed foods often contain additives and preservatives that may disrupt thyroid function. These additives can contain synthetic colors, flavors, and preservatives that could potentially disrupt hormonal balance and impact overall well-being. Opting for whole, unprocessed foods can help steer clear of these detrimental substances.

Caffeine and Alcohol

Both caffeine and alcohol have the potential to disrupt thyroid function and worsen symptoms of hypothyroidism. It is important to exercise moderation when dealing with these substances.

Excessive caffeine intake can disrupt sleep patterns and cause adrenal stress, which can have a negative impact on thyroid health. However, moderate caffeine consumption can still be incorporated into a healthy diet. Caffeine has the ability to stimulate the adrenal glands, leading to the production of stress hormones. This, in turn, can disrupt the delicate equilibrium of thyroid hormones. Limiting caffeine consumption, particularly in the later parts of the day, can have a positive impact on thyroid health and enhance the quality of sleep.

Alcohol has the potential to disrupt the production and metabolism of thyroid hormones. In addition, the liver can be impacted as it plays a crucial role in converting T4 to the active T3 hormone. Excessive alcohol consumption can disrupt the conversion process, resulting in imbalances in thyroid hormone levels. Optimizing thyroid health can be achieved by stopping alcohol consumption or limiting its intake.

Understanding the importance of diet in maintaining optimal thyroid health is crucial, as it has a significant impact on hormone production, immune function, and overall well-being. With a deep understanding of the nutrients necessary for optimal thyroid function and by making well-informed dietary choices, individuals with hypothyroidism have the power to greatly improve their overall health. Including iodine-rich seafood, selenium-packed nuts, zinc and iron from lean meats, and a variety of fruits and vegetables in your diet, while limiting or avoiding the consumption of goitrogenic foods, gluten, processed foods, and excessive caffeine and alcohol can help maintain thyroid function and promote overall health.

4.2. Dietary Plans

Developing a dietary plan that promotes optimal thyroid health goes beyond simply selecting appropriate foods. Having a well-thought-out strategy for meal planning, considering nutrient timing, and gaining knowledge about the impact of various foods on thyroid function is crucial. This subchapter offers a range of dietary plans specifically designed to support individuals with hypothyroidism. It includes detailed meal plans and recipes that aim to optimize thyroid function and promote overall well-being.

For optimal thyroid health, it's important to prioritize a well-balanced diet that includes nutrient-rich foods packed with vital vitamins and minerals, while steering clear of any that may disrupt thyroid function. Here, we will discuss the key elements of a well-rounded dietary plan, covering breakfast, lunch, dinner, and snacks.

Breakfast: Starting the Day Right

Nutrient Goals: Focus on protein, healthy fats, and complex carbohydrates to stabilize blood sugar levels and provide sustained energy throughout the morning. Ensure a good intake of iodine, selenium, and other essential nutrients.

Sample Breakfast Plan

1) Scrambled Eggs with Spinach and Mushrooms

Ingredients:
- 3 large eggs
- 1 cup fresh spinach
- 1/2 cup sliced mushrooms
- 1/4 cup diced onions
- 1 tbsp olive oil
- Salt and pepper to taste

Preparation:

1. Heat olive oil in a pan over medium heat. Add onions and sauté until translucent.
2. Add mushrooms and spinach, cooking until the spinach is wilted and mushrooms are tender.
3. Beat the eggs in a bowl, season with salt and pepper, and pour into the pan. Stir continuously until the eggs are fully cooked.

This breakfast provides a balanced mix of protein, healthy fats, and fiber, alongside essential nutrients like selenium from the eggs and antioxidants from the vegetables.

2) Vegetable Omelette with Avocado

Ingredients:
- 3 large eggs
- 1/4 cup diced bell peppers
- 1/4 cup diced onions
- 1/4 cup chopped spinach
- 1/4 cup sliced mushrooms
- 1 avocado, sliced
- 1 tbsp olive oil
- Salt and pepper to taste

Preparation:

1. Heat olive oil in a pan over medium heat. Add bell peppers, onions, spinach, and mushrooms. Sauté until vegetables are tender.
2. Beat the eggs in a bowl, season with salt and pepper, and pour into the pan with the vegetables.
3. Cook until the eggs are set, folding the omelette in half. Serve with sliced avocado on the side.

This omelette is packed with protein, healthy fats, and a variety of vitamins and minerals to start your day on the right foot.

3) Greek Yogurt Parfait

Ingredients:
  - 1 cup Greek yogurt
  - 1/2 cup mixed berries (blueberries, strawberries, raspberries)
  - 1/4 cup granola (low sugar)
  - 1 tbsp honey
  - 1 tbsp chia seeds

Preparation:

1. Layer Greek yogurt, mixed berries, and granola in a bowl or jar.
2. Drizzle with honey and sprinkle with chia seeds.
3. Enjoy a protein-packed, antioxidant-rich start to your day.

4) Banana and Nut Butter Smoothie

Ingredients:
  - 1 banana
  - 1 cup almond milk
  - 2 tbsp almond butter
  - 1 tbsp chia seeds
  - 1/2 tsp cinnamon
  - 1 cup ice cubes

Preparation:

1. Combine all ingredients in a blender and blend until smooth.
2. Pour into a glass and enjoy a nutritious and energizing smoothie.

Lunch: Midday Nutrient Boost

Nutrient Goals: Incorporate lean proteins, a variety of vegetables, and whole grains. Include foods rich in zinc and iron to support thyroid hormone synthesis and overall energy levels.

Sample Lunch Plan

1) Grilled Chicken Salad with Quinoa and Avocado

Ingredients:
    - 1 grilled chicken breast, sliced
    - 1 cup cooked quinoa
    - 1/2 avocado, sliced
    - 1 cup mixed greens (spinach, kale, arugula)
    - 1/2 cup cherry tomatoes, halved
    - 1/4 cup sliced cucumbers
    - 1/4 cup shredded carrots
    - 2 tbsp olive oil

- 1 tbsp balsamic vinegar
- Salt and pepper to taste

Preparation:

1. Cook quinoa according to package instructions and let cool.
2. In a large bowl, combine mixed greens, cherry tomatoes, cucumbers, and shredded carrots.
3. Add sliced grilled chicken, quinoa, and avocado.
4. Drizzle with olive oil and balsamic vinegar, then toss to combine.
5. Season with salt and pepper to taste.

This salad is rich in protein, healthy fats, and a variety of vitamins and minerals. The quinoa and mixed greens provide carbs and other essential nutrients, while the avocado adds healthy fats to help with nutrient absorption.

2) Turkey and Avocado Wrap

Ingredients:
- 1 rice tortilla
- 4 slices of turkey breast
- 1/2 avocado, sliced
- 1/2 cup mixed greens (lettuce, spinach, arugula)
- 1/4 cup shredded carrots
- 2 tbsp hummus
- Salt and pepper to taste

Preparation:

1. Spread hummus evenly over the rice tortilla.
2. Layer turkey slices, avocado, mixed greens, and shredded carrots on top of the hummus.
3. Season with salt and pepper.
4. Roll up the tortilla tightly and slice in half.

This wrap provides a balanced mix of protein, healthy fats, and fiber, making it a satisfying and nutritious lunch option.

3) Shrimp and Avocado Salad

Ingredients:
- 1 lb cooked shrimp, peeled and deveined
- 2 avocados, diced
- 1 cup cherry tomatoes, halved
- 1/4 cup red onion, finely chopped
- 1/4 cup fresh cilantro, chopped
- Juice of 1 lime
- 2 tbsp olive oil
- Salt and pepper to taste

Preparation:

1. In a large bowl, combine shrimp, avocados, cherry tomatoes, red onion, and cilantro.
2. In a small bowl, whisk together lime juice, olive oil, salt, and pepper.
3. Pour the dressing over the salad and toss gently to com-

bine.

4. Serve immediately or chill for 30 minutes for flavors to meld.

4) Salmon and Avocado Salad

Ingredients:
- 1 grilled salmon fillet, flaked
- 1 avocado, sliced
- 2 cups mixed greens
- 1/2 cup cherry tomatoes, halved
- 1/4 cup cucumber, sliced
- 2 tbsp olive oil
- 1 tbsp lemon juice
- Salt and pepper to taste

Preparation:

1. Combine mixed greens, cherry tomatoes, and cucumber in a bowl.
2. Add flaked salmon and sliced avocado.
3. Drizzle with olive oil and lemon juice, then toss to combine.
4. Season with salt and pepper to taste.

Dinner: Nourishing and Satisfying

Nutrient Goals: Focus on a balanced meal that includes lean proteins, vegetables, and healthy fats. Ensure the inclusion of foods that support thyroid health, such as seafood for iodine and selenium.

Sample Dinner Plan

1) Baked Salmon with Asparagus and Sweet Potatoes

Ingredients:
- 1 salmon fillet (about 6 oz)
- 1 bunch of asparagus, trimmed
- 1 large sweet potato, cubed
- 2 tbsp olive oil
- 1 lemon, sliced
- 2 cloves garlic, minced
- Salt, pepper, and fresh dill to taste

Preparation:

1. Preheat the oven to 400°F (200°C).
2. Place the salmon fillet on a baking sheet lined with parchment paper. Drizzle with olive oil, and top with minced garlic, lemon slices, and fresh dill. Season with salt and pepper.
3. Arrange the asparagus and sweet potato cubes around the

salmon. Drizzle with the remaining olive oil and season with salt and pepper.

4. Bake in the preheated oven for 20–25 minutes, or until the salmon is fully cooked and the vegetables are tender.
5. Serve immediately, garnished with additional lemon slices if desired.

This dinner is nutrient-dense and packed with omega-3 fatty acids from the salmon, fiber, and vitamins from the vegetables. Sweet potatoes provide a good source of complex carbohydrates and antioxidants.

2) Beef Stir-Fry with Zucchini and Bell Peppers

Ingredients:
   - 1 lb lean beef sirloin, thinly sliced
   - 2 cups zucchinis
   - 1 cup sliced bell peppers
   - 1/2 cup sliced onions
   - 2 cloves garlic, minced
   - 2 tbsp soy sauce (low sodium)
   - 1 tbsp sesame oil
   - 1 tbsp olive oil
   - 1 tsp grated ginger
   - 1 cup cooked rice

Preparation:

1. Heat olive oil in a large pan or wok over medium-high heat. Add garlic and ginger, sautéing until fragrant.

2. Add sliced beef and cook until browned.
3. Add zucchinis, bell peppers, and onions, stirring frequently until vegetables are tender-crisp.
4. Stir in soy sauce and sesame oil, mixing well to combine.
5. Serve over cooked rice.

This stir-fry is a delicious and nutrient-dense dinner option, offering lean protein, fiber, and a variety of vitamins and minerals.

3) Herb-Crusted Cod with Rice and Asparagus

Ingredients:
  - 2 cod fillets
  - 1 cup rice
  - 1 bunch asparagus, trimmed
  - 2 tbsp olive oil
  - 2 tbsp fresh parsley, chopped
  - 1 lemon, sliced
  - 2 cloves garlic, minced
  - Salt and pepper to taste

Preparation:

1. Preheat the oven to 400°F (200°C).
2. Cook rice according to package instructions and set aside.
3. Place cod fillets on a baking sheet lined with parchment paper. Drizzle with olive oil, sprinkle with minced garlic, parsley, salt, and pepper. Top with lemon slices.
4. Arrange asparagus around the cod and drizzle with olive

oil. Season with salt and pepper.

5. Bake for 20-25 minutes until the cod is cooked through and the asparagus is tender.
6. Serve the cod and asparagus with a side of rice.

4) Pork Tenderloin with Roasted Vegetables

Ingredients:
- 1 pork tenderloin
- 2 zuchinis, sliced
- 2 carrots, sliced
- 1 red onion, quartered
- 2 tbsp olive oil
- 1 tbsp fresh rosemary, chopped
- 2 cloves garlic, minced
- Salt and pepper to taste

Preparation:

1. Preheat the oven to 400°F (200°C).
2. Rub the pork tenderloin with olive oil, garlic, rosemary, salt, and pepper.
3. Arrange zucchini, carrots, and red onion around the tenderloin on a baking sheet.
4. Drizzle the vegetables with olive oil and season with salt and pepper.
5. Roast in the oven for 25-30 minutes, or until the pork is cooked through and the vegetables are tender.
6. Slice the pork and serve with roasted vegetables.

Snacks: Keeping Energy Levels Stable

Nutrient Goals: Choose snacks that provide a steady source of energy and essential nutrients without causing blood sugar spikes. Include options rich in fiber, healthy fats, and protein.

Sample Snack Ideas

1) Greek Yogurt with Nuts and Berries

Ingredients:
  - 1 cup Greek yogurt
  - 1/4 cup mixed nuts (almonds, Brazilian nuts, walnuts, cashews)
  - 1/2 cup fresh berries (blueberries, strawberries, raspberries)
  - 1 tsp honey (optional)

Preparation:

1. Combine Greek yogurt, mixed nuts, and fresh berries in a bowl.
2. Drizzle with honey if desired.
3. Enjoy as a protein-packed, nutrient-rich snack.

2) Apple Slices with Almond Butter

Ingredients:
  - 1 apple, sliced
  - 2 tbsp almond butter

Preparation:

  1. Core and slice the apple.
  2. Spread almond butter on each apple slice.
  3. Enjoy a snack that provides healthy fats, protein, and fiber.

3) Carrot and Celery Sticks with Hummus

Ingredients:
  - 2 carrots, peeled and cut into sticks
  - 2 celery stalks, cut into sticks
  - 1/4 cup hummus

Preparation:
   1. Serve carrot and celery sticks with a side of hummus for a crunchy and nutritious snack.

4) Snack: Almonds and Orange Slices

Ingredients:
  - 1 orange, sliced
  - 1/4 cup almonds

Preparation:

1. Slice the orange and serve with a handful of almonds for a nutritious and satisfying snack.

Integrating Nutrient Timing and Meal Frequency

In addition to choosing the right foods, paying attention to nutrient timing and meal frequency can enhance thyroid function and overall energy levels.

Consistent Meal Timing

Eating meals at regular intervals helps maintain stable blood sugar levels and prevents energy dips. Aim for three main meals and possibly two snacks per day, ensuring that each eating occasion includes a balance of macronutrients.

Pre- and Post-Workout Nutrition

For those who exercise regularly, incorporating pre-and post-workout nutrition can support energy levels and recovery. A small snack with protein and carbohydrates before exercise can fuel the workout, while a post-workout meal or snack with protein and healthy fats can aid in muscle repair and replenishment.

Hydration

Staying hydrated is essential for overall health and metabolic function. Aim to drink at least eight 8-ounce glasses of water per day, adjusting for activity level and climate. Herbal teas and water-rich foods like fruits and vegetables can also contribute to hydration.

Additional Recipes for Thyroid Health

Recipe 1: Lemon Herb Grilled Chicken

Ingredients:
- 4 boneless, skinless chicken breasts
- 1/4 cup olive oil
- Juice of 2 lemons
- 4 cloves garlic, minced
- 1 tbsp fresh rosemary, chopped
- 1 tbsp fresh thyme, chopped
- Salt and pepper to taste

Preparation:

1. In a bowl, mix olive oil, lemon juice, garlic, rosemary, thyme, salt, and pepper.
2. Add chicken breasts to the marinade and let sit for at least 30 minutes.
3. Preheat grill to medium-high heat.
4. Grill chicken breasts for 6-7 minutes per side, or until

fully cooked.
5. Serve with a side of roasted vegetables or a fresh salad.

Recipe 2: Beef and Sweet Potato Skillet

Ingredients:
 - 1 lb lean ground beef
 - 1 large sweet potato, peeled and diced
 - 1 bell pepper, diced
 - 1 onion, diced
 - 2 cloves garlic, minced
 - 2 tbsp olive oil
 - 1 tsp paprika
 - 1 tsp cumin
 - Salt and pepper to taste
 - Fresh parsley for garnish

Preparation:

1. Heat olive oil in a large skillet over medium heat. Add onion and garlic, cooking until translucent.
2. Add ground beef, cooking until browned and crumbled. Drain excess fat.
3. Add sweet potato, bell pepper, paprika, cumin, salt, and pepper. Stir to combine.
4. Cover and cook for 10–15 minutes, stirring occasionally, until sweet potatoes are tender.
5. Garnish with fresh parsley and serve hot.

Recipe 3: Herb-Roasted Chicken with Root Vegetables

Ingredients:
- 1 whole chicken (3-4 lbs)
- 4 carrots, peeled and chopped
- 3 parsnips, peeled and chopped
- 1 onion, quartered
- 4 cloves garlic, minced
- 2 tbsp olive oil
- 1 tbsp fresh rosemary, chopped
- 1 tbsp fresh thyme, chopped
- Salt and pepper to taste

Preparation:

1. Preheat oven to 375°F (190°C).
2. In a roasting pan, toss carrots, parsnips, and onion with olive oil, garlic, rosemary, thyme, salt, and pepper.
3. Place chicken on top of the vegetables and season generously with salt and pepper.
4. Roast for 1 hour 30 minutes, or until the chicken reaches an internal temperature of 165°F (75°C).
5. Let the chicken rest for 10 minutes before carving. Serve with roasted vegetables.

Recipe 4: Baked Cod with Tomato and Basil

Ingredients:
- 4 cod fillets

- 2 cups cherry tomatoes, halved
- 1/4 cup fresh basil, chopped
- 2 cloves garlic, minced
- 2 tbsp olive oil
- Juice of 1 lemon
- Salt and pepper to taste

Preparation:

1. Preheat oven to 400°F (200°C).
2. In a baking dish, arrange cod fillets and surround with cherry tomatoes.
3. In a small bowl, mix olive oil, lemon juice, garlic, salt, and pepper.
4. Pour the mixture over the cod and tomatoes.
5. Bake for 20 minutes or until the cod is cooked through and flakes easily with a fork.
6. Sprinkle with fresh basil before serving.

Recipe 5: Grilled Chicken and Avocado Salad

Ingredients:
- 1 grilled chicken breast, sliced
- 1 avocado, sliced
- 2 cups mixed greens (spinach, kale, arugula)
- 1/2 cup cherry tomatoes, halved
- 1/4 cup cucumber, sliced
- 1/4 cup red onion, thinly sliced

- 2 tbsp olive oil
- 1 tbsp balsamic vinegar
- Salt and pepper to taste

Preparation:

1. Combine mixed greens, cherry tomatoes, cucumber, and red onion in a large bowl.
2. Add sliced grilled chicken and avocado.
3. Drizzle with olive oil and balsamic vinegar, then toss to combine.
4. Season with salt and pepper to taste.

Recipe 6: Turkey Lettuce Wraps

Ingredients:
- 4 large lettuce leaves (romaine or butter lettuce)
- 8 slices of turkey breast
- 1/2 avocado, sliced
- 1/2 cup shredded carrots
- 1/4 cup red bell pepper, sliced
- 2 tbsp hummus
- Salt and pepper to taste

Preparation:

1. Spread hummus on each lettuce leaf.
2. Layer turkey slices, avocado, shredded carrots, and bell pepper.

3. Season with salt and pepper, then roll up the lettuce leaves to form wraps.

Additional Breakfast Recipes

Spinach and Parmesan Cheese Omelette

Ingredients:
- 3 large eggs
- 1 cup fresh spinach, chopped
- 1/4 cup parmesan cheese, crumbled (better if aged 36 months)
- 1/4 cup diced tomatoes
- 1 tbsp olive oil
- Salt and pepper to taste

Preparation:

1. Heat olive oil in a pan over medium heat. Add spinach and cook until wilted.
2. Beat eggs in a bowl, season with salt and pepper, and pour into the pan.
3. Add diced tomatoes and parmesan cheese on one side of the omelette.
4. Cook until eggs are set, then fold the omelette in half and serve.

Spinach and Mushroom Frittata

Ingredients:
- 6 large eggs
- 1 cup fresh spinach, chopped
- 1 cup mushrooms, sliced
- 1/2 cup diced onions
- 1/2 cup parmesan cheese, crumbled
- 2 tbsp olive oil
- Salt and pepper to taste

Preparation:

1. Preheat the oven to 350°F (175°C).
2. Heat olive oil in an oven-safe skillet over medium heat. Add onions and mushrooms, sautéing until tender.
3. Add spinach and cook until wilted.
4. In a bowl, beat the eggs and season with salt and pepper.
5. Pour the eggs into the skillet and cook for a few minutes until the edges start to set.
6. Sprinkle parmesan cheese over the top and transfer the skillet to the oven.
7. Bake for 10-15 minutes, or until the frittata is fully set and golden brown.
8. Slice and serve warm.

These recipes are designed to support thyroid health by incorporating nutrient-dense ingredients that provide essential vitamins and minerals while avoiding foods that may interfere with thyroid function. Enjoy these meals as part of a balanced diet to help manage hypothyroidism and promote overall well-being.

Conclusion

In conclusion, the relationship between diet and thyroid health is profound and multifaceted. The thyroid gland relies on specific nutrients to function optimally, and dietary choices can either support or hinder this delicate balance. Through careful selection of nutrient-rich foods and mindful eating habits, individuals with hypothyroidism can significantly influence their thyroid function and overall health.

The dietary plans and recipes provided in this chapter offer practical guidance for incorporating essential nutrients such as iodine, selenium, zinc, iron, vitamin D, omega-3 fatty acids, and B vitamins into daily meals. These nutrients play critical roles in thyroid hormone synthesis, immune modulation, and metabolic regulation. By prioritizing foods that enhance thyroid health and avoiding those that interfere with thyroid function, individuals can create a supportive dietary environment conducive to managing hypothyroidism.

Moreover, understanding the importance of nutrient timing, meal frequency, and hydration further enhances the effectiveness of dietary interventions. Consistent meal timing helps stabilize blood sugar levels, while proper hydration supports metabolic processes and overall well-being. Pre- and post-workout nutrition can also aid in energy management and recovery, particularly for those with active lifestyles.

By taking control of their dietary choices and embracing a nutrient-rich lifestyle, individuals with hypothyroidism can empower themselves to achieve better symptom control, enhanced energy levels, and improved quality of life. This chapter aims to equip readers with the knowledge and tools necessary to make informed dietary decisions, fostering a proactive and health-conscious approach to thyroid management.

5

Managing Symptoms

"Health is not just about what you're eating. It's also about what you're thinking and saying."

This quote encapsulates the holistic approach necessary for managing hypothyroidism—a condition that affects not only the body but also the mind. Managing the symptoms of hypothyroidism is a complex task that requires more than just medication. While hormone replacement therapy is essential, addressing the broader lifestyle factors that influence symptom management is equally critical.

In this chapter, we explore the multifaceted strategies necessary for effectively managing the symptoms of hypothyroidism. We delve into the importance of environmental factors like air and water quality, which can subtly but significantly impact thyroid health. We also examine the role of sleep hygiene in supporting cognitive function and overall well-being, emphasizing the need for quality rest in mitigating the effects of brain fog and fatigue. Additionally, this chapter focuses on mental health and well-being, offering insights into coping with cognitive symptoms and employing stress management techniques. These strategies are not just about alleviating symptoms but about empowering individuals to take control of their health and improve their quality of life.

5.1. Lifestyle Factors that Influence Thyroid Health

Thyroid health is impacted by various factors that extend beyond medical treatments and diet. Although these elements are essential, there are other lifestyle factors that can greatly affect thyroid function and overall well-being. This subchapter delves into the impact of environmental toxins, sleep hygiene, and lifestyle choices on thyroid health. It provides practical strategies to enhance resilience and promote overall well-being.

Environmental Toxins and Their Impact on Thyroid Health

Understanding the impact of the environment on our health is vital, especially for those dealing with hypothyroidism. Being mindful of how specific environmental factors can affect thyroid function is key. The thyroid gland is highly susceptible to toxins that can interfere with hormone production and regulation. Having a good grasp of these potential risks and being proactive in minimizing exposure can go a long way in safeguarding thyroid health.

Exposure to plastics and chemicals in our daily lives is almost impossible to avoid completely. However, there are certain compounds, like bisphenol A (BPA) and phthalates, that are especially worrisome when it comes to thyroid health. These chemicals are classified as endocrine disruptors, which can disrupt the normal hormonal balance in the body, including the hormones produced by the thyroid gland.

Bisphenol A (BPA)

BPA is a frequently encountered substance in plastic containers, water bottles, and the lining of canned foods. It has the potential to seep into food and beverages, particularly when plastics are heated, like in a microwave. Once inside the body, BPA has the ability to imitate or interfere with hormone signals, which can potentially result in thyroid dysfunction. Studies have indicated a link between BPA exposure and changes in thyroid hormone levels, potentially worsening conditions such as hypothyroidism.

Phthalates

Phthalates are commonly found in various products, including personal care items like shampoos and lotions, as well as household items such as vinyl flooring and plastic toys. Similar to BPA, phthalates have the potential to disrupt hormone function by interfering with the body's endocrine system. Research has established a connection between elevated phthalate levels and disruptions in thyroid hormone levels, which can have repercussions on metabolism and overall well-being.

Minimizing Contact

To minimize your contact with these potentially harmful substances, take into account the following approaches:

- Opt for products that are free of BPA, particularly when it comes to storing food and beverages.

- It is advisable to refrain from using plastic containers for microwaving food.

- Choose glass, stainless steel, or other materials that are considered safer for storing food and beverages.

Make sure to read the labels on personal care products and opt for options that do not contain phthalates. It is advisable to reduce the usage of plastics, particularly in items that have direct contact with food or beverages.

Heavy Metals

It is important to be aware of the presence of heavy metals such as mercury and lead in the environment, as they have the potential to build up in the body and cause a range of health problems, including thyroid dysfunction. These metals can disrupt the thyroid's hormone production, resulting in various symptoms linked to hypothyroidism.

Mercury

Mercury is a harmful metal that can be found in specific fish species, dental amalgams, and industrial pollution. It has the potential to build up in the body, especially in the thyroid gland, disrupting the production of hormones. Research has established a connection between mercury exposure and autoimmune thyroiditis.

Lead

Exposure to lead, which can occur through various sources such as old paint, contaminated water, and specific industrial processes, can have detrimental effects on thyroid health. Lead can interfere with the production and regulation of thyroid hormones, resulting in imbalances that contribute to the symptoms of hypothyroidism.

Minimizing Contact

To reduce your risk of heavy metal exposure, you may want to consider taking the following steps:

- It is advisable to reduce the intake of high-mercury fish, including shark, swordfish, and king mackerel. Instead, choose seafood with lower mercury levels such as salmon, shrimp, and catfish.

- It is advisable to have a conversation with your dentist regarding the safe removal options for dental amalgams.

Make sure to check your home and water supply for any potential lead contamination, especially if you reside in an older house.

Air and Water Quality

Understanding the importance of clean air and water for our well-being, it becomes evident that these factors play a key role in maintaining optimal thyroid function. Having a clear understanding of the link between environmental quality and thyroid health is crucial for individuals dealing with conditions such as hypothyroidism. Even small changes in the environment can have a significant impact on symptom management and overall well-being.

Air Quality

Air pollution poses a significant but often unnoticed danger to the health of the thyroid. Environmental pollutants can have a significant impact on the thyroid gland, leading to oxidative stress and inflammation in the body. Stress can have a negative impact on the thyroid's hormone production and regulation, which can worsen symptoms for those with hypothyroidism.

Urban environments carry specific risks due to their elevated levels of industrial emissions, vehicle exhaust, and particulate matter. These pollutants contain heavy metals and chemical compounds that have the potential to disrupt the endocrine system. It is important to note that particulate matter, composed of minuscule particles suspended in the air, has the ability to deeply infiltrate the lungs and enter the bloodstream. This can have a significant impact on various organs and glands in the body, such as the thyroid. Research has indicated that prolonged exposure to air pollution is linked to a higher likelihood of developing thyroid disorders, specifically autoimmune thyroiditis.

Aside from industrial pollutants, indoor air quality is also a matter of concern. Household products like cleaning agents, paints, and furniture can release volatile organic compounds (VOCs) that can accumulate in poorly ventilated spaces. This can result in a harmful build-up of chemicals in the home. These compounds have the potential to disturb the delicate balance of hormones, placing additional strain on the thyroid gland.

Addressing the impacts of subpar air quality necessitates a combination of knowledge and proactive measures. Using air purifiers that filter out pollutants, allergens, and VOCs is a highly effective method for enhancing indoor air quality. Properly ventilating living spaces through the strategic use of windows and exhaust fans can effectively decrease the presence of indoor pollutants. For individuals residing in heavily polluted urban areas, it can be beneficial to limit time spent outdoors on days with high pollution levels and to wear masks that can filter out particulate matter. These measures can contribute to safeguarding thyroid health.

Water quality

Water is essential for the proper functioning of every cell and organ in the body, including the thyroid gland. Nevertheless, the water's quality can vary greatly, and if it becomes contaminated, it can negatively impact thyroid health. Understanding the thyroid's dependence on iodine is crucial for the production of vital hormones. Nevertheless, the equilibrium can be disturbed by impurities that are frequently present in drinking water.

Fluoride and Chlorine

Fluoride and chlorine are frequently included in municipal water supplies to safeguard dental health and eliminate harmful bacteria. Nevertheless, both of these substances can disrupt thyroid function. Fluoride, specifically, has a chemical resemblance to iodine and can potentially interfere with its absorption by the thyroid gland. This competition may result in a decrease in iodine availability, which can negatively impact thyroid hormone production and potentially worsen symptoms of hypothyroidism.

Although chlorine is necessary for ensuring the safety of water supplies, it can also have negative effects on thyroid health. When chlorine reacts with organic matter in water, it produces by-products called trihalomethanes (THMs), which have been associated with several health concerns, including possible disruptions to thyroid function. In addition, chlorine has the potential to remove essential minerals from water, which can lead to dehydration and have a negative impact on one's overall well-being.

Concerns about heavy metals and other contaminants

Besides fluoride and chlorine, drinking water may contain heavy metals like lead, mercury, and arsenic. These metals have been identified as disruptors of the endocrine system and can build up in the body over time, resulting in various health problems, such as thyroid dysfunction. Lead has been linked to a reduced thyroid hormone production, while mercury can disrupt the function of the thyroid gland by binding to it.

Additional pollutants, like pesticides and industrial chemicals, may enter the water supply via agricultural runoff or industrial waste. These chemicals have the ability to imitate or hinder hormones, causing disruptions in the endocrine system and potentially leading to thyroid issues.

Enhancing Water Quality

It is essential to prioritize the quality of the water you consume in order to safeguard your thyroid health. Using a top-notch water filtration system is a highly effective method for enhancing water quality. It can eliminate chlorine, fluoride, heavy metals, and various other impurities. There are different types of filters to choose from, such as activated carbon filters that effectively eliminate chlorine and VOCs, or reverse osmosis systems that can remove a wider range of contaminants, including fluoride and heavy metals.

Aside from filtration, it is important to consider the origin of your water. If you reside in an area where water quality concerns are prevalent, such as excessive industrial pollution or agricultural runoff, it may be prudent to take extra measures. This could involve opting for bottled water for drinking and cooking purposes.

Regularly testing your water for contaminants can give you peace of mind and help you confirm that your filtration system is working effectively. You can easily find home water testing kits that can identify various common contaminants, enabling you to address any issues that may arise.

Sleep Hygiene

Sleep is a vital aspect of overall well-being, yet it is frequently overlooked. Having proper sleep is essential for individuals with hypothyroidism, as it is crucial for their well-being. The thyroid gland has a huge role in the body's sleep-wake cycle, as it regulates metabolism and energy levels. Effective sleep hygiene helps manage symptoms of hypothyroidism, including fatigue, cognitive dysfunction, and mood disturbances. Poor sleep can worsen these symptoms, so it's important to prioritize good sleep habits.

The Link Between Thyroid Function and Sleep

The connection between thyroid health and sleep goes both ways. Individuals with hypothyroidism commonly experience symptoms such as fatigue, sluggishness, and depression, which can significantly affect their sleep patterns. On the other hand, inadequate sleep can also worsen the functioning of the thyroid. For example, insufficient sleep has been proven to impact the body's stress response, resulting in higher cortisol levels. This can disrupt the production of thyroid hormones and worsen symptoms of hypothyroidism.

In addition, sleep plays a crucial role in the body's natural repair processes, which include regulating hormones. While we sleep, our body diligently works to restore and balance hormone levels, including the thyroid. Insufficient sleep can seriously disrupt these processes, exacerbating the symptoms of hypothyroidism. Prioritizing good sleep hygiene is absolutely essential for individuals managing thyroid disorders.

Creating the Perfect Sleep Environment

Creating an environment that promotes rest is essential for maintaining good sleep hygiene. Your bedroom should be a tranquil heaven, a place where you can unwind and let go of all the worries and tensions of the day. An optimal sleep environment requires a cool and comfortable room temperature, usually ranging from 60-67 degrees Fahrenheit. It's important to acknowledge the significance of darkness, as exposure to light can disrupt the production of melatonin, the hormone responsible for regulating sleep. Creating a dark environment can be achieved by using blackout curtains, eye masks, or simply turning off all lights and electronic devices.

Excessive noise can also disturb sleep, therefore it is crucial to reduce any disturbances. Using white noise machines, earplugs, or even a fan can effectively minimize external sounds. In addition, it's important to make sure that the mattress and pillows provide comfort and support, as this can greatly impact the quality of sleep. For individuals dealing with hypothyroidism, who may experience muscle and joint pain, it is important to consider investing in a top-notch mattress that promotes proper body alignment. This can provide significant benefits.

Maintaining a regular sleep routine is key for good sleep hygiene. Maintaining a consistent sleep schedule, even on weekends, is crucial for regulating the body's internal clock, also known as the circadian rhythm. This regularity facilitates a more seamless transition into sleep and awakening, thereby minimizing the chances of experiencing sleep disorders such as insomnia.

Establishing a pre-sleep routine can effectively signal to the body that it's time to relax and prepare for rest. This routine could involve activities such as reading, indulging in a soothing bath, or engaging in relaxation techniques like deep breathing or meditation. It is important to refrain from engaging in stimulating activities before going to bed, such as vigorous exercise or consuming caffeine. Instead, try engaging in soothing activities that encourage relaxation and help prepare your body for a restful night's sleep.

Reducing the use of screens before bedtime is an essential aspect of maintaining good sleep habits. Exposure to the blue light emitted by phones, tablets, and computers can disrupt the production of melatonin, which can make it more difficult to fall asleep. It is recommended to turn off all screens at least an hour before bedtime. If you find yourself in a situation where using screens is necessary, there are options available to help reduce the negative impact. Blue light filters or glasses can be quite effective in mitigating the effects.

The Relationship Between Nutrition and Sleep

Your sleep quality can be greatly influenced by the food and beverages you consume throughout the day. Avoiding heavy, rich, or spicy meals near bedtime can help prevent discomfort and indigestion, which can disrupt sleep. It is recommended to complete your meals at least two to three hours before bedtime.

Certain foods, on the other hand, can contribute to improved sleep. Consuming foods that are high in tryptophan, like turkey, dairy products, and nuts, can help boost serotonin levels, which then gets converted into melatonin. In the same way, complex carbohydrates can enhance the availability of tryptophan in the brain, which helps promote better sleep. Herbal teas, like chamomile or valerian root, have soothing properties that promote relaxation before bedtime.

Managing Stress and Relaxation Techniques

Stress often plays a significant role in disrupting sleep patterns, particularly for those with hypothyroidism, who may already be grappling with feelings of anxiety or depression. Incorporating stress management techniques into your daily routine can effectively decrease your overall stress levels, allowing for a more relaxed evening wind-down. Practices such as mindfulness meditation, yoga, and progressive muscle relaxation can be highly effective.

Keeping a journal before going to sleep can be a highly effective technique. Jotting down thoughts, concerns, or to-do items for the following day can be beneficial in decluttering the mind, minimizing the inclination to dwell on them while in bed. For certain individuals, utilizing guided imagery or listening to calming music or nature sounds can foster a peaceful mental state that promotes better sleep.

The Importance of Physical Activity

Engaging in regular physical activity can have a positive impact on sleep patterns. However, it's important to consider the timing and intensity of your exercise routine as they can influence the quality of your sleep. Participating in moderate aerobic exercise, like walking or swimming, can assist in achieving faster sleep onset and experiencing more restful sleep. On the other hand, engaging in intense physical activity right before going to bed can actually have a counterproductive outcome, as it may leave you feeling too alert and energized to fall asleep. It is recommended to finish intense workouts at least three hours prior to going to bed.

Practicing yoga and engaging in stretching exercises, particularly in the evening, can help induce a sense of calmness and prime the body for a restful night's sleep. Engaging in gentle stretching can effectively alleviate muscle tension, while practicing yoga has been shown to effectively reduce stress and promote a sense of calmness. Even a brief evening yoga routine can have a positive impact on the quality of your sleep.

If sleep issues continue despite following proper sleep hygiene practices, it might be advisable to consider consulting a professional. A healthcare provider has the ability to screen for sleep disorders, including sleep apnea, which tends to be more prevalent in individuals with hypothyroidism. CBT-I is a proven treatment method that effectively targets chronic sleep problems by modifying thoughts and behaviors related to sleep.

Optimizing thyroid hormone levels is crucial for improving sleep in individuals with hypothyroidism. Consistently seeking guidance from a healthcare professional to closely monitor and make necessary adjustments to medication can have a notable impact on the quality of sleep.

Environmental factors, including exposure to toxins and poor air and water quality, can significantly affect thyroid health, often worsening the symptoms of hypothyroidism. By implementing measures to minimize contact with potentially harmful substances and enhancing the overall quality of your living space, you can effectively promote the health of your thyroid and enhance your overall sense of well-being. In order to effectively manage hypothyroidism, it is crucial to prioritize sleep hygiene. Getting enough sleep is crucial for hormone regulation and overall thyroid health. It allows the body to repair and rejuvenate, contributing to a holistic approach to maintaining thyroid health. By making conscious decisions about their lifestyle and cultivating a nurturing atmosphere, people with hypothyroidism can enhance their ability to bounce back and enhance their overall well-being.

5.2. Mental Health and Well-being

Living with hypothyroidism can be a complex journey, involving both physical symptoms and the mental and emotional hurdles that accompany the condition. Experiencing cognitive symptoms like brain fog, memory lapses, and difficulty concentrating can be incredibly challenging, affecting one's daily life and overall sense of well-being. In addition, the stress and anxiety that come with managing a chronic illness can worsen these symptoms, creating a challenging cycle to overcome. This section explores effective techniques for dealing with cognitive symptoms and handling stress, providing practical tips to improve mental health and overall well-being.

Dealing with Cognitive Symptoms

Individuals with hypothyroidism often experience cognitive symptoms, commonly known as "brain fog." These symptoms may manifest as challenges in memory, focus, and cognitive processing, resulting in feelings of frustration and reduced efficiency. Gaining insight into the root causes of these symptoms and devising effective strategies to manage them is crucial for enhancing one's quality of life.

Exploring Brain Fog

Brain fog is not a term commonly used in the medical field, but it is often used to describe various cognitive issues that can impact the clarity of one's thoughts. Brain fog in hypothyroidism is commonly associated with the disruption of thyroid hormones, which have a significant impact on brain function.

Insufficient levels of thyroid hormones can have a negative impact on cognitive functions, resulting in challenges with focus, recall, and critical thinking.

It is worth noting that hypothyroidism can disrupt the balance of hormones in the body, leading to changes in neurotransmitter levels in the brain. Specifically, serotonin and dopamine, which play a big role in regulating mood and cognitive function, may be impacted. This disturbance can lead to sensations of bewilderment, memory lapses, and an overall perception of cognitive lethargy.

Stress Management Techniques

Mastering stress management is important for individuals with hypothyroidism, as it requires a delicate balance of art and science. Chronic stress has the potential to worsen symptoms, disturb hormone balance, and contribute to a cycle of physical and mental health difficulties. With the proper strategies, one can successfully navigate through the challenges of stress and come out stronger, more focused, and with improved overall well-being.

Stress is a common reaction to perceived threats, a remnant of our evolutionary history where it played a vital role in ensuring survival. In today's society, the stress response can be activated by various situations that are not necessarily life-threatening, such as work deadlines, financial concerns, or even traffic jams. For individuals with hypothyroidism, managing stress becomes even more important due to the body's heightened response to stress. It is essential to develop effective strategies for stress management.

When stress is encountered, the body's fight-or-flight response is triggered. This response is controlled by the release of hormones like adrenaline and cortisol, which prime the body to either confront or escape from danger. Although this response can be helpful in small doses, long-term activation of the stress response can result in various health problems, such as compromised thyroid function.

Cortisol, commonly known as the "stress hormone," has a significant impact on thyroid health. When present in limited quantities, cortisol helps maintain a balanced metabolism and bolstering the immune system. Extended exposure to elevated cortisol levels can hinder the conversion of T4 to T3, which is essential for optimal thyroid function. This suppression can worsen symptoms of hypothyroidism, including fatigue, weight gain, and depression.

The Power of Breath: Embracing Inner Serenity

Deep breathing is a highly effective stress management technique that can be easily practiced. The breath is an incredibly powerful tool that has the ability to swiftly transition the body from a state of stress to one of deep relaxation. During times of stress, our breathing tends to become shallow and rapid, which sends a signal to the body that it is in a state of danger.

By intentionally slowing down and deepening your breath, you can signal to your nervous system that it's okay to unwind and relax.

Deep breathing stimulates the parasympathetic nervous system, which is commonly referred to as the "rest and digest" system. This system works to counteract the fight-or-flight response, resulting in a decrease in heart rate, a reduction in blood pressure, and the promotion of a state of tranquility. Practicing techniques like diaphragmatic breathing, which involves deep belly breaths instead of shallow chest breaths, can be done anytime and anywhere. By simply dedicating a few moments to centering your attention on your breath, you can effectively transform your stress levels.

Movement as Medicine: The Role of Exercise in Stress Relief

Engaging in regular physical activity can be a powerful way to manage stress. Regular exercise has a multitude of benefits for both the body and mind. It improves cardiovascular health, builds strength, and enhances flexibility, while also having profound effects on mental well-being. Engaging in physical activity triggers the release of endorphins, which are the brain's natural "feel-good" chemicals. Endorphins play a crucial role in reducing stress, enhancing mood, and promoting a sense of well-being.

For individuals dealing with hypothyroidism, fatigue and sluggishness can pose significant challenges, making the idea of exercise appear overwhelming. However, it's important to discover types of exercise that you genuinely enjoy and can maintain over time.

The Healing Power of Connection: Building a Support Network

As social beings, humans rely on connections with others to effectively manage stress. Having a strong network of friends and loved ones can greatly help in mitigating the negative impact of stress. Engaging in conversations with loved ones, bonding with family members, or joining a support group can offer a deep sense of connection, affirmation, and empathy.

For people with hypothyroidism, who may feel isolated or misunderstood, discovering a supportive community can be life-changing. Consider joining a local or online support group where you can connect with others who have faced similar experiences, challenges, and triumphs. Understanding that there are others who share your journey can bring great solace and alleviate the emotional weight of managing a long-term condition.

In addition, engaging in acts of kindness and assisting others can also serve as a means of alleviating stress. Research has demonstrated that engaging in selfless acts can effectively alleviate stress and enhance one's overall sense of happiness and well-being. Engaging in acts of kindness, whether it's through volunteering, assisting a neighbor, or offering words of encouragement, can create a positive cycle that improves both your own well-being and that of others.

The Transformative Power of Mindfulness and Meditation for Optimal Thyroid Health

Mindfulness and meditation hold significant value in today's wellness culture, extending beyond mere trendy terms. These practices have a rich history in ancient traditions and provide substantial advantages for mental, emotional, and physical well-being. For individuals with hypothyroidism, where stress and cognitive challenges such as brain fog are common, these practices can provide significant benefits. Practicing mindfulness and meditation can be incredibly beneficial for managing the mental and emotional symptoms that often accompany thyroid disorders. These techniques offer valuable tools to calm the mind, reduce stress, and enhance overall well-being.

Mindfulness involves fully focusing on the present moment, embracing curiosity and acceptance. One aspect of this practice is to simply observe thoughts, feelings, and sensations as they arise, without any judgment or the need to alter them. This approach enables individuals to develop a heightened awareness of their internal experiences, enabling them to respond to situations with enhanced clarity and composure, rather than reacting impulsively or out of habit.

For individuals dealing with hypothyroidism, the symptoms can be quite overwhelming and intrusive. However, practicing mindfulness can provide a valuable tool for regaining control and gaining a fresh perspective. Through the practice of mindfulness, people can develop the ability to calmly observe their symptoms, such as fatigue, brain fog, or anxiety, without being overwhelmed by them. Approaching the situation from a different angle can help lessen the emotional impact of symptoms and allow for more deliberate and controlled reactions to the difficulties of managing a long-term condition.

Meditation is an essential component of mindfulness practice, requiring the mind to concentrate on a specific object, thought, or activity in order to attain mental clarity and emotional serenity. Studies have indicated that consistent meditation can result in alterations to the brain's structure, specifically in regions linked to focus, recall, and managing stress.

It has been widely observed in neuroscience that meditation has the potential to enhance the thickness of the prefrontal cortex, which helps in executive functions like decision-making, problem-solving, and emotional regulation. For individuals with hypothyroidism, who may experience cognitive symptoms, these changes can be especially helpful.

In addition, studies have demonstrated that meditation can decrease the size and activity of the amygdala, which is the part of the brain responsible for fear responses. This decrease in levels can help alleviate the anxiety and stress commonly experienced by individuals with thyroid conditions. Meditation has been found to have a positive impact on cortisol levels, which can in turn benefit both mental and physical well-being. By calming the amygdala, meditation helps to reduce the levels of this stress hormone, which is known to interfere with thyroid function.

Practical Methods for Embracing Mindfulness and Meditation

Integrating mindfulness and meditation into your daily routine doesn't necessitate lengthy, intensive sessions. Consistent daily practice, no matter how brief, can lead to noticeable advantages. Here's how you can incorporate these practices into your daily routine if you're managing hypothyroidism:

Morning Mindfulness Practice: Begin your day with a straight-forward mindfulness exercise to cultivate a sense of presence and awareness. As you wake up, take a moment to pay attention to your breath, the sensation of your body on the bed, and any thoughts or emotions that arise. This routine establishes a serene and concentrated atmosphere for the day, aiding in the management of stress right from the beginning.

Practicing Meditative Breathing: Incorporate moments of calm into your daily routine, particularly during times of stress or when symptoms become more pronounced. Dedicate a few minutes to centering yourself and paying attention to your breath. Take a moment to close your eyes, breathe in deeply through your nose, hold for a brief pause, and then exhale slowly through your mouth. This easy breathing technique is highly effective in reducing stress and promoting a deep sense of calm.

Beginner's Meditation: If you're new to meditation, guided meditations can be a great way to get started. There are plenty of apps and online resources available that provide guided sessions tailored to help reduce stress, enhance focus, and promote overall well-being. These sessions come in different lengths, so you can easily find one that suits your schedule.

Body Scan Meditation: This form of meditation guides you through a thorough examination of your body, helping you become aware of any areas of tension or discomfort. It is especially beneficial for individuals with hypothyroidism, as they may encounter muscle pain or fatigue. By highlighting these areas, you can alleviate tension and encourage relaxation.

Evening Reflection: Conclude your day with a short meditation or mindfulness exercise. Take a moment to contemplate the events of the day, paying attention to any thoughts or emotions that may still be present, without passing any judgment. This technique promotes mental clarity, facilitating easier sleep and ensuring a more rejuvenating night.

The Long-Term Benefits of Mindfulness and Meditation

Mindfulness and meditation offer a wide range of benefits that go beyond simply relieving stress. With consistent application, these practices can bring about significant transformations in your perception of symptoms, your physical well-being, and your overall quality of life.

Regular meditation can improve emotional resilience, making it easier to handle the challenges of living with hypothyroidism. It promotes a feeling of tranquility and balance, even when dealing with physical discomfort or mental confusion. This strength is not only about persevering through difficulties, but about flourishing in spite of them—discovering moments of happiness, appreciation, and satisfaction even in the face of ongoing symptoms.

Mindfulness also helps foster self-compassion, a crucial trait for individuals dealing with a long-term condition. Through the practice of mindfulness, one can cultivate a compassionate and non-judgmental attitude towards oneself, fostering kindness and understanding instead of frustration or self-criticism. Embracing this change in mindset can greatly enhance your mental and emotional health, alleviating the psychological toll of hypothyroidism.

Discover the Calming Effects of Nature: How the Outdoors Can Help Reduce Stress

Immersing oneself in the great outdoors can be highly beneficial for reducing stress and regaining a feeling of equilibrium. Being in nature can have a soothing impact on both the mind and body, offering a respite from the never-ending stimulation of our fast-paced world. Spending time in nature, whether it's strolling through a park, trekking up a mountain, or just relaxing by a lake, provides an opportunity to unwind, take in fresh air, and reestablish a connection with the environment.

Studies have demonstrated that being in natural environments can effectively decrease cortisol levels, lower blood pressure, and enhance overall mood. Spending time in the forest, according to research, has been shown to have remarkable benefits in reducing stress and enhancing immune function. Spending time in any natural setting, whether it's a garden, a beach, or even your backyard, can provide similar benefits, even if you don't live near a forest.

Immersing oneself in nature provides a tranquil setting to cultivate mindfulness. Immersing oneself in the beauty of nature can enhance mindfulness and promote a sense of calm, allowing for a release of stress and concerns.

The Art of Saying No: Establishing Boundaries to Safeguard Your Well-being

Mastering the art of stress management requires the ability to establish boundaries and confidently decline requests when appropriate. For many individuals, the constant expectations from others, be it at work, in social settings, or within the family, can result in long-term stress and exhaustion. For individuals with hypothyroidism, who may already feel overwhelmed by the demands of managing their condition, this holds especially true.

Establishing boundaries requires acknowledging your personal limitations and effectively conveying them to others. This could involve prioritizing self-care, managing work responsibilities, and being selective with social commitments. Declining certain requests is essential for your own self-care, enabling you to prioritize your health and overall well-being.

Practicing assertiveness and self-compassion are crucial for establishing healthy boundaries. Expressing your needs and desires confidently and respectfully is an important aspect of assertiveness. It is equally important to treat yourself with kindness and understanding, especially during times when you may be feeling overwhelmed.

Embracing Relaxation: Adding Downtime to Your Daily Schedule

It is key to include regular downtime in your routine to effectively manage stress and maintain balance. In our fast-paced society, finding moments to relax and unwind can be seen as unproductive or even self-indulgent. However, finding time to relax is not a luxury; it is essential for maintaining good mental and physical health.

Resting is essential for both your physical and mental well-being, enabling your body and mind to rejuvenate after the demands of everyday life. Engaging in various activities like reading, listening to music, practicing yoga, or enjoying a warm bath can be beneficial. It's important to discover activities that promote relaxation and rejuvenation, enabling you to approach your obligations with a fresh sense of vitality and concentration.

Understanding the importance of mental health and well-being is crucial for effectively managing hypothyroidism. Dealing with cognitive symptoms such as brain fog necessitates making lifestyle changes and implementing support strategies that can improve cognitive function and alleviate frustration. Implementing a range of stress management techniques, such as deep breathing, physical activity, mindfulness, and meditation, can effectively reduce the negative effects of stress on thyroid health and enhance overall well-being.

Developing emotional resilience through cultivating a positive mindset, embracing self-compassion, and honing problem-solving skills is essential for effectively navigating the complexities of life.

Conclusion

Managing the symptoms of hypothyroidism requires a holistic approach that considers both the physical and mental aspects of health. Throughout this chapter, we have explored various strategies that extend beyond traditional medical treatments, highlighting the importance of environmental awareness, sleep hygiene, and stress management in supporting thyroid function and overall well-being.

By understanding the impact of environmental toxins, indi-

viduals can make informed choices to reduce exposure and protect their thyroid health. Prioritizing sleep and incorporating mindfulness practices can help alleviate cognitive symptoms, improving focus and reducing the pervasive fatigue that often accompanies hypothyroidism. Stress management, through techniques such as deep breathing, physical activity, and building strong social connections, plays a huge role in mitigating the harmful effects of chronic stress on the thyroid and the body as a whole.

Ultimately, managing hypothyroidism is about more than just addressing symptoms as they arise; it's about creating a supportive environment—both internally and externally—that fosters long-term health and resilience. By embracing these strategies, individuals can take proactive steps toward managing their condition, improving their quality of life, and living well with hypothyroidism.

6

Long-Term Management and Lifestyle

"Success is the sum of small efforts, repeated day in and day out."

This quote by Robert Collier perfectly encapsulates the approach required to effectively manage hypothyroidism over the long term. Hypothyroidism isn't a condition that can be solved with a one-time fix; it demands ongoing attention, lifestyle adjustments, and a commitment to health that integrates into your daily life. This chapter explores the essential elements of long-term management and lifestyle strategies that can significantly impact your health journey with hypothyroidism.

In this chapter, we discuss the importance of regular monitoring and follow-up to ensure that your thyroid function remains stable and your treatment effective. We also delve into the critical role of physical exercise, which not only supports a healthy metabolism but also enhances overall physical and mental health. Through regular exercise, individuals can counteract the weight gain, fatigue, and muscle weakness commonly associated with hypothyroidism. This chapter offers practical insights into how these strategies can be integrated into your life, helping you to maintain balance, improve your quality of life, and effectively manage hypothyroidism for the long haul.

6.1. Monitoring and Follow-up

Managing hypothyroidism is a lifelong journey that demands continuous attention, not only in terms of treatment but also through regular monitoring and follow-up. Beginning thyroid hormone replacement therapy (THRT) is an essential part of managing hypothyroidism, but it's important to remember that the process doesn't stop there. Consistent monitoring, timely adjustments, and close collaboration with your health-care provider are crucial for ensuring the effectiveness of treatment and maintaining the stability of your thyroid function. This section delves into the significance of regular testing, comprehending the timing and reasons for adjustments, and the role of actively collaborating with your healthcare team.

The Importance of Regular Testing

Hypothyroidism is a condition characterized by the thyroid gland's inability to produce sufficient amounts of thyroid hormones, specifically thyroxine (T4) and triiodothyronine (T3). Regular testing is necessary to monitor hormone levels and ensure they are within the optimal range, ever since the introduction of thyroid hormone replacement therapy (THRT).

Regular blood tests, usually measuring levels of Thyroid Stimulating Hormone (TSH), are essential for monitoring thyroid function. TSH is produced by the pituitary gland and instructs the thyroid to increase its production of T4 and T3. Typically, in cases of hypothyroidism, TSH levels tend to be elevated as the body attempts to encourage the underactive thyroid to generate more hormones. THRT aims to bring TSH levels back within a normal range, and ongoing monitoring is necessary to achieve this goal.

Testing is essential as the body's requirements may vary over time. Various factors, including the natural aging process, fluctuations in weight, pregnancy, stress, and alterations in diet or medication, can impact the body's utilization of thyroid hormones. Regular testing is crucial to account for these variables and make timely adjustments to THRT.

Healthcare providers typically advise patients to undergo TSH level testing every six to twelve months, depending on the stability of their condition. Additionally, it may be important to consider more frequent testing during periods of significant change, such as when initiating or modifying medication, throughout pregnancy, or when symptoms resurface after a period of stability.

Your healthcare provider may also keep an eye on free T4 and free T3 levels, especially if there are concerns that TSH alone may not provide a complete picture of your thyroid status. Measuring the levels of Free T4 and T3 can offer valuable insights into the availability of thyroid hormone for your cells, which can aid in refining your treatment.

It is often necessary to make adjustments to your medication regimen when managing hypothyroidism. Thyroid hormone requirements can vary over time, and what may be effective for you at one stage of your life may not be as beneficial in the future. Regular monitoring and follow-up are crucial in ensuring proper adjustment.

Recognizing the Necessity for Adjustment

Thyroid medication adjustments are usually determined by analyzing blood test results and considering the symptoms experienced. Even if your TSH levels fall within the normal range, it is possible to experience symptoms that indicate a need for dose adjustment. If you experience persistent fatigue, weight gain, hair loss, depression, or difficulty concentrating, it could be a sign that adjustments are needed. On the other hand, symptoms such as anxiety, insomnia, or unexplained weight loss may suggest an overactive thyroid.

Occasionally, modifications may be required due to changes in your lifestyle and overall health. For instance, substantial changes in weight can impact your thyroid hormone requirements. During pregnancy, it is important to closely monitor thyroid hormone levels and potentially adjust the dosage to promote the well-being of both the mother and the baby.

When a modification is necessary, your healthcare provider will usually suggest a slight adjustment in your thyroid hormone dosage, followed by another round of testing in six to eight weeks. This waiting period is essential as it allows the body sufficient time to adjust to the medication change and for the TSH level to reach a stable state.

The objective of any adjustment is to discover the ideal equilibrium where symptoms are effectively managed and hormone levels are within an optimal range. It's a journey that demands patience and meticulous observation of your body's response to every adjustment. Sometimes, it might require multiple adjustments to determine the optimal dosage.

Collaborating with Your Healthcare Provider

Managing hypothyroidism requires a collaborative approach, where you and your healthcare provider work together to achieve optimal results. This partnership is founded on transparent communication, a strong sense of trust, and a shared dedication to monitoring and follow-up.

When it comes to selecting a healthcare provider, it's important to make an informed decision. Finding a professional who is experienced and knowledgeable in their field is paramount. Take the time to research and consider various factors before making your choice. Your health is too important to leave in the hands of someone who may not have the expertise you need. Trust your instincts and seek out a healthcare provider who is well-respected and trusted in their profession.

It is crucial to have a healthcare provider who is well-versed in thyroid disorders. With their specialized knowledge in hormone-related conditions, including hypothyroidism, endocrinologists are able to provide expert guidance. It's important to find a healthcare professional who values your input, respects your symptoms, and actively monitors your condition.

Mastering the art of effective communication is key in any professional setting. It is essential to convey information clearly and concisely, ensuring that your message is understood by all parties involved. By honing your communication skills, you can foster strong relationships, resolve conflicts, and achieve your goals with ease.

Having open and clear communication with your healthcare provider is essential for effectively managing your health. It is important to be open and transparent about your symptoms, even if they may appear insignificant, and to communicate any alterations in your well-being or daily routine that could potentially impact your thyroid function. If you're experiencing symptoms that indicate your medication may need adjustment, feel free to discuss them during your appointments. Your input is fundamental in assisting your provider in making well-informed decisions regarding your care.

It's important to have a conversation about any other medications or supplements you're currently using, as they may have interactions with thyroid hormone replacement therapy. Take note that the absorption of thyroid medication can be disrupted if calcium and iron supplements are taken too closely together. Additionally, it's important to be aware that thyroid hormone levels can be influenced by certain medications used to treat conditions such as heart disease or diabetes.

Maintaining a health diary or utilizing a tracking app can prove to be a valuable method for monitoring various aspects of your well-being, such as symptoms, energy levels, mood, and other factors that may be impacted by your thyroid function. Having this information available during your appointments can give your healthcare provider a more comprehensive understanding of how your treatment is progressing and identify any necessary adjustments.

Make sure to schedule regular follow-up appointments and don't hesitate to contact your healthcare provider if you experience any notable changes in your symptoms between visits. Early intervention is crucial in preventing minor issues from escalating into major problems.

Living with hypothyroidism can be a lifelong journey, with unexpected challenges that may arise along the way. Your healthcare provider is there to support you in managing the impact of aging on your thyroid function, dealing with other health conditions that complicate treatment, or navigating the emotional toll of a chronic illness. This enduring partnership is founded on a shared sense of respect and a dedication to adjusting your treatment as necessary throughout the course of your journey.

Collaborating with a healthcare provider is essential, but it's equally important to take charge of your own health when managing hypothyroidism in the long run. Having knowledge about your condition, comprehending your treatment choices, and actively engaging in your care are all elements of self-advocacy that can result in improved health outcomes.

Having a good grasp of the fundamentals of hypothyroidism and its treatment allows you to make well-informed choices regarding your healthcare. Having this knowledge allows for a better understanding of the significance of regular testing, the ability to identify signs that medication adjustments may be necessary, and the confidence to ask pertinent questions during appointments.

Feel free to ask any questions if you need clarification about your treatment. Your healthcare provider is available to address any questions or concerns you may have regarding the frequency of testing, the implications of your test results, or the side effects of your medication. When you ask questions, it demonstrates your commitment to understanding your treatment and taking an active role in your health management.

If you're feeling dissatisfied with the care you're receiving or if you're facing complex issues that haven't been resolved, seeking a second opinion can be a valuable step. Another health-care provider may provide a different viewpoint or recommend alternative treatment options that could potentially be more beneficial for you.

Managing hypothyroidism is an ever-evolving process that demands continuous attention and adjustment. With the proper approach and support, it is completely feasible to lead a fulfilling life with this condition, ensuring equilibrium, well-being, and energy in the long run.

6.2. The Role of Exercise in Hypothyroidism Management

Regular exercise is essential for individuals with hypothyroidism to effectively manage their condition and improve overall well-being. Individuals with an underactive thyroid gland experience a range of physical and mental difficulties. These may include weight gain, fatigue, muscle weakness, and a sluggish metabolism. Incorporating regular exercise into your daily routine is a highly effective method to combat these symptoms and enhance your overall well-being in the long run.

Exploring the Link Between Hypothyroidism and Exercise

Having an underactive thyroid can greatly impact metabolism, making it challenging to manage weight and causing ongoing fatigue and lack of energy. Regular physical activity is crucial in countering these effects as it boosts the metabolism, increases energy levels, and promotes overall well-being.

Individuals with hypothyroidism often struggle with a slowed metabolism, which can result in weight gain and challenges in losing weight. Engaging in regular exercise, particularly aerobic activities such as walking, running, cycling, and swimming, can effectively combat the metabolic slowdown. Engaging in these activities can help elevate your heart rate, burn calories, and optimize energy utilization. This is particularly important for weight management if you have a slower metabolism caused by hypothyroidism.

Engaging in regular aerobic exercise can greatly enhance cardiovascular health, which is especially crucial considering the heightened susceptibility to heart disease linked to hypothyroidism. Through its positive impact on heart and lung function, exercise helps the body process oxygen and nutrients more effectively, resulting in increased metabolic rate and energy levels.

Building Muscle Through Strength Training

Strength training is especially advantageous for individuals with hypothyroidism, in addition to aerobic exercise. Increasing muscle mass can significantly boost your basal metabolic rate (BMR), as muscle tissue burns more calories than fat, even at rest. Strength training exercises, such as weightlifting, resistance band workouts, and bodyweight exercises like squats and push-ups, are important for maintaining muscle mass and supporting a healthy metabolism.

Strength training provides a range of benefits for individuals with hypothyroidism, extending beyond just metabolism. Improving bone density is vital due to the potential for hypothyroidism to weaken bones. Additionally, it improves joint stability and overall strength, which lowers the chances of getting injured and facilitates participation in various physical activities.

Boosting Energy Levels and Combating Fatigue

Fatigue is a prevalent and incapacitating symptom of hypothyroidism. Contrary to common belief, exercise is actually a highly effective method for combating fatigue. Engaging in regular physical activity can boost the production of endorphins, the body's natural mood enhancers. This can lead to improved energy levels and a decrease in feelings of fatigue.

Regular exercise helps regulate the body's energy production systems, making it more convenient to carry out daily tasks and alleviating the persistent fatigue commonly associated with hypothyroidism. With regular physical activity, individuals can gradually build up their stamina and endurance, allowing them to fully participate in various work and personal activities.

Enhancing Flexibility and Promoting Joint Health

It is important to incorporate flexibility and balance exercises into your routine as hypothyroidism can cause joint pain, stiffness, and decreased mobility. Practices like yoga and Pilates offer great benefits as they emphasize stretching, strengthening, and balancing the body. Engaging in these activities can help enhance flexibility, range of motion, muscle strength, and joint health.

Yoga, especially, provides the additional advantage of including mindfulness and relaxation techniques, which can aid in reducing stress, a well-known trigger for hypothyroid symptoms. Practicing yoga and Pilates can have a positive impact on your body. The gentle movements and deep breathing techniques can help alleviate muscle and joint tension, decrease inflammation, and enhance blood flow. These benefits can ultimately lead to improved mobility and reduced pain.

Mental Health Benefits

In addition to its physical advantages, consistent exercise plays a vital role in promoting mental well-being, which is particularly important for individuals with hypothyroidism who may be more susceptible to feelings of depression and anxiety. Engaging in physical activity triggers the release of neurotransmitters that regulate mood, such as serotonin and dopamine. Exercise has been found to boost the production of certain chemicals in the body that are associated with positive emotions. This can lead to a reduction in symptoms of depression and anxiety, offering a natural and effective method for enhancing mental well-being.

In addition, following a consistent exercise regimen can help foster a feeling of achievement and direction, crucial for sustaining an optimistic mindset and countering the cognitive haze and fatigue commonly linked to hypothyroidism. Participating in group activities, like fitness classes or walking groups, can also strengthen social connections, which in turn promotes emotional well-being.

Customizing Exercise for Personal Requirements

It is critical to customize your physical activity based on your specific needs and current health condition, particularly if you are dealing with hypothyroidism. Although the advantages of exercise are evident, it is essential to take into account your individual circumstances. It is better to start off slowly and gradually increase the intensity and duration of workouts, especially for individuals who are new to exercise or have been inactive for a while.

Engaging in low-impact activities like walking, swimming, or using an elliptical machine can serve as an excellent foundation for improving fitness levels while minimizing stress on the joints. As you continue to improve your fitness, you can gradually introduce more demanding exercises into your routine, such as interval training, higher-intensity cardio, or advanced strength training workouts.

It is essential to pay close attention to your body. Include rest days in your exercise routine and be mindful of how your body reacts to various forms of exercise, as hypothyroidism may hinder your recovery from intense physical activity.

To achieve lasting success in managing hypothyroidism, it is key to incorporate exercise into your daily routine in a manner that is both sustainable and enjoyable. Discovering activities that bring you joy, like dancing, hiking, or cycling, can be a great way to incorporate movement into your daily routine. You can also make small changes, such as opting for the stairs instead of the elevator or walking instead of driving for short distances.

Establishing attainable objectives and monitoring your advancement can also assist in sustaining motivation and guaranteeing that you're adhering to your fitness regimen. Tracking your progress, whether through a fitness app, workout journal, or simply noting how you feel after each workout, can give you a sense of accomplishment and motivate you to continue.

The Long-Term Effects of Regular Exercise

Regular exercise offers a wide range of benefits that go well beyond its immediate impact on metabolism, energy levels, and mental well-being. Consistent physical activity can bring about remarkable improvements in overall health and quality of life over time. Regular exercise help individuals with hypothyroidism to prevent the long-term complications linked to the condition, including heart disease, osteoporosis, and insulin resistance.

In addition, integrating exercise into your daily routine establishes a solid basis for a healthier and more active lifestyle, which promotes both your physical and mental well-being. Exercise transforms from a mere symptom management tool into a lifestyle that boosts your overall well-being, contentment, and satisfaction.

Conclusion

The long-term management of hypothyroidism is a dynamic, ongoing process that requires consistency, adaptation, and a proactive approach to health. As we've explored in this chapter, managing hypothyroidism effectively involves more than just taking medication; it requires a comprehensive strategy that includes regular monitoring, exercise, and lifestyle adjustments tailored to your individual needs.

Regular follow-up appointments and testing ensure that your treatment remains effective and responsive to changes in your body. Coupled with this medical vigilance, integrating exercise into your routine plays a pivotal role in combating the metabolic slowdowns, weight gain, and fatigue often associated with hypothyroidism. Exercise is not merely a physical activity but a powerful tool for enhancing mental clarity, mood, and overall resilience.

By focusing on these key areas—monitoring, exercise, and lifestyle—you create a robust foundation for long-term health and well-being. The consistency of these efforts, repeated day in and day out, helps you navigate the complexities of hypothyroidism with confidence and grace, enabling you to lead a full, active, and healthy life despite the challenges of a chronic condition. The strategies outlined in this chapter are designed to empower you, helping you take control of your health and live well with hypothyroidism for years to come.

7

Special Considerations

"Health is a state of complete harmony of the body, mind, and spirit."

This quote by B.K.S. Iyengar underscores the importance of a holistic approach to managing hypothyroidism, particularly when it intersects with other life stages and conditions. Hypothyroidism is not a one-size-fits-all condition; it presents unique challenges at different stages of life and often coexists with other health issues that complicate its management. Understanding these special considerations is crucial for providing comprehensive care that addresses the full spectrum of a patient's health needs.

In this chapter, we explore the complexities of hypothyroidism as it manifests in various life stages—children, adolescents, pregnancy, and postpartum—and how it interacts with other health conditions. These discussions highlight the importance of tailored treatment approaches that consider the unique physiological and psychological demands at each stage of life. We also examine the challenges posed by co-existing conditions such as autoimmune disorders and other health issues that frequently accompany hypothyroidism. By delving into these special considerations, this chapter aims to equip patients with the knowledge necessary to manage hypothyroidism effectively in the context of broader health challenges.

7.1. Hypothyroidism in Different Life Stages

Hypothyroidism can present differently at different stages of life, making it a complex condition to understand. Throughout different stages of life, from childhood to pregnancy and postpartum, the effects of an underactive thyroid can vary greatly. This requires personalized approaches to diagnosing, treating, and managing the condition. Having a comprehensive understanding of how hypothyroidism manifests and impacts individuals at various stages of life is essential for providing effective care and ensuring a high quality of life. This subchapter delves into the intricacies of hypothyroidism in children, adolescents, and women during pregnancy and the postpartum period, providing valuable insights into the unique challenges and factors to consider at each stage.

Hypothyroidism in Children and Adolescents

Managing hypothyroidism in children and adolescents can pose distinct challenges that have a profound impact on a young individual's growth, development, and overall well-being. In contrast to adults, where the focus is mainly on maintaining energy levels and metabolic function, hypothyroidism in younger individuals can disrupt important processes such as physical growth, brain development, and emotional regulation. It is of utmost importance to address hypothyroidism in children and adolescents as early as possible in order to maximize their physical and mental development.

The Effects on Growth and Development

The thyroid hormone is crucial for maintaining proper growth and development of the body. For children, bone growth and brain development are of utmost importance. When a child experiences hypothyroidism, the insufficiency of thyroid hormones can result in various developmental challenges.

Untreated hypothyroidism in children can lead to stunted growth, which is a cause for concern. During puberty, the growth plates in a child's bones close, allowing for a limited window of opportunity for growth. If hypothyroidism goes undetected and untreated, it can lead to delayed bone growth, resulting in a shorter stature and delayed puberty. Children diagnosed with hypothyroidism may also face challenges in their mental development, potentially impacting their academic performance and cognitive abilities.

In addition to supporting physical growth, thyroid hormones play a vital role in the development of the brain. In infants and young children, hypothyroidism can result in cretinism, which is characterized by significant intellectual disabilities, motor skill deficits, and hearing issues. Even a slight case of hypothyroidism in older children can lead to challenges in learning, problems with memory, and a shorter attention span.

Recognizing Symptoms in Children and Adolescents

Identifying hypothyroidism in children and adolescents can pose a challenge as the symptoms are often subtle and can be confused with typical developmental changes or other health concerns. It is crucial for parents and healthcare providers to remain attentive in recognizing potential indicators of thyroid dysfunction.

Infants with congenital hypothyroidism may exhibit symptoms such as prolonged jaundice, an enlarged tongue, weak muscle tone, and challenges with feeding. As the child develops, delayed milestones, such as walking or talking later than expected, can also be signs to consider.

For older children and adolescents, symptoms may appear as fatigue, weight gain even with normal or reduced food intake, dry skin, constipation, and sensitivity to cold. Adolescents may also encounter delayed puberty, irregular menstrual cycles, and mood swings, which can add complexity to the diagnosis. Regular monitoring of thyroid function is crucial, particularly if there is a family history of thyroid disease, as these symptoms can often be mistakenly attributed to other causes.

The Importance of Early Diagnosis

Early detection of hypothyroidism in children and adolescents is vital in order to prevent potential long-term complications. As part of routine newborn screening programs, hypothyroidism is commonly screened for in many countries. Early detection of congenital hypothyroidism enables timely treatment, preventing the occurrence of significant cognitive and developmental delays.

On the other hand, hypothyroidism may also manifest in later stages of childhood or adolescence. Autoimmune thyroiditis, also referred to as Hashimoto's thyroiditis, is a prevalent cause of hypothyroidism in older children and adolescents. This condition occurs when the immune system mistakenly attacks the thyroid gland, resulting in a decrease in hormone production.

Regular health check-ups are essential for closely monitoring a child's growth and development, allowing for early detection of hypothyroidism. If there are any concerns regarding a child's growth rate, cognitive development, or the presence of other symptoms that may indicate thyroid dysfunction, a straightforward blood test can be conducted to measure levels of Thyroid Stimulating Hormone (TSH) and thyroxine (T4) in order to confirm the diagnosis.

Treatment and Management

Once diagnosed, the treatment for hypothyroidism in children and adolescents is quite simple. The main course of treatment involves thyroid hormone replacement therapy, usually with levothyroxine, a synthetic version of T4. The objective of treatment is to achieve balanced thyroid hormone levels, enabling the child to experience normal growth and development.

The dosage of thyroid hormone replacement therapy is meticulously determined, taking into account the child's weight, age, and the extent of the hypothyroidism. Since children are still growing, their medication needs may change frequently. It is important to have regular follow-up appointments to monitor TSH and T4 levels and make any necessary adjustments to the dosage.

Typically, children diagnosed with hypothyroidism will require lifelong thyroid hormone replacement therapy. With appropriate treatment, individuals can live healthy, ordinary lives with minimal, if any, restrictions. Parents and caregivers must prioritize the consistent administration of medication to children and be aware that even small gaps in treatment can result in the reemergence of symptoms.

Addressing the Psychological and Emotional Impact

Not only do children and adolescents with hypothyroidism experience physical symptoms, but they may also face significant psychological and emotional effects. Experiencing fatigue, struggling to concentrate, and dealing with mood swings can all have a negative impact on a child's academic and social performance. These challenges can be especially difficult during adolescence, a period when teenagers are already navigating the complexities of self-discovery, social dynamics, and academic achievement.

For teenagers, the physical changes linked to hypothyroidism can pose significant challenges, including weight gain and delayed puberty. Dealing with body image concerns, along with the emotional rollercoaster of hypothyroidism, can contribute to feelings of low self-worth, heightened anxiety, and depression.

Recognizing and addressing psychological and emotional challenges is crucial for parents, caregivers, and healthcare providers. Some children and adolescents may find counseling or therapy helpful in managing the emotional aspects of hypothyroidism. Support groups, whether they are held in person or online, can offer a valuable sense of community and empathy for young individuals managing the condition.

The Long-term Outlook

With early diagnosis and appropriate treatment, the long-term prognosis for children and adolescents with hypothyroidism is typically quite favorable. Many individuals can experience normal growth and development, reach their maximum potential in academics and extracurricular pursuits, and lead a vibrant and healthy lifestyle.

It is important to keep in mind that hypothyroidism is a condition that needs continuous management throughout one's life. As kids mature and make their way into adulthood, they'll have to shoulder greater responsibility for handling their condition. It is essential to educate children and adolescents about their thyroid health, the significance of taking medication as prescribed, and how to identify symptoms of thyroid dysfunction. This knowledge empowers them to manage their health as they grow older.

Hypothyroidism During Pregnancy and Postpartum

During pregnancy, there are significant changes that occur, not only on an emotional and physical level, but also in terms of hormonal fluctuations. Managing these changes for women with hypothyroidism can be particularly intricate, necessitating meticulous care to safeguard the well-being of both the mother and the developing baby. Dealing with hypothyroidism during pregnancy can have major consequences, and the postpartum period presents its own unique set of difficulties. Having a good grasp of how to navigate these stages with hypothyroidism is essential for the health and happiness of both the mother and child.

The Role of Thyroid Hormones in Pregnancy

Thyroid hormones play a critical role in the proper development of a fetus, especially in the early stages of pregnancy when the baby's own thyroid gland is not fully operational. Throughout this stage, the developing fetus depends solely on the thyroid hormones produced by the mother. These hormones play a vital role in the growth of the brain, nervous system, and overall physical development. During pregnancy, the need for thyroid hormones rises, which can put extra strain on the mother's thyroid gland.

Meeting the increased demand can be challenging for women with hypothyroidism, where the thyroid gland is already un-deractive. When hypothyroidism is not effectively treated during pregnancy, it can result in various complications such as miscarriage, preterm birth, low birth weight, and develop-mental delays in the baby. In addition, if hypothyroidism in the mother is left untreated, it can raise the chances of developing preeclampsia, a serious condition that involves high blood pressure and harm to various organs.

Diagnosing and Managing Hypothyroidism during Pregnancy

Given the crucial importance of thyroid hormones during pregnancy, it is imperative to diagnose and manage hypothyroidism early on. It is recommended that women with known hypothyroidism undergo thyroid function testing before conception or as soon as they discover their pregnancy. Healthcare providers can make early treatment adjustments to accommodate the heightened hormonal demands of pregnancy.

Management usually requires adjusting the dosage of thyroid hormone replacement therapy, typically levothyroxine, in order to maintain optimal thyroid hormone levels. It is essential to regularly monitor the body's thyroid hormone needs during pregnancy, as they can vary. It is recommended by the American Thyroid Association to monitor thyroid function regularly throughout pregnancy, with more frequent checks during the first half and at least one check during the second half. Regular check-ups are important to ensure the well-being of both the mother and the baby during their development.

Understanding the connection between thyroid hormone levels and pregnancy outcomes is of utmost importance. Even when TSH levels are elevated but T4 levels remain within the normal range, untreated subclinical hypothyroidism can lead to negative outcomes. It is essential to prioritize maintaining tight control over thyroid hormone levels during pregnancy.

The Relationship Between Hypothyroidism and Fertility

It's worth mentioning that hypothyroidism can also have an impact on fertility. Women who have untreated or poorly managed hypothyroidism may face challenges when trying to conceive because their menstrual cycles and ovulation can be disrupted. Thyroid hormones have a strong connection to reproductive hormones, and when there are imbalances, it can result in anovulation (failure to ovulate) or irregular periods, which can decrease the likelihood of conception.

It is important for women with hypothyroidism who are planning to become pregnant to have their thyroid function evaluated and optimized before attempting to conceive. Proper pre-pregnancy management can enhance fertility and minimize the chances of complications during pregnancy.

The Impact of Hypothyroidism on Labor and Delivery

Hypothyroidism can have an impact on the process of labor and delivery. Women who have poorly controlled hypothyroidism face a greater likelihood of encountering complications during childbirth, such as prolonged labor or the necessity for a cesarean section. There are several factors to consider here: muscle weakness caused by hypothyroidism can potentially hinder the efficiency of uterine contractions during labor. In addition, thyroid hormones also contribute to the production of oxytocin, a hormone that is crucial for the progression of labor. If there is a lack of thyroid hormone levels, it can result in low oxytocin levels, which can then lead to ineffective labor contractions.

In addition, women with hypothyroidism have a higher risk of experiencing postpartum hemorrhage, which is characterized by excessive bleeding after childbirth. It is believed that this is connected to the decrease in muscle tone and slower blood clotting times that are commonly seen in individuals with thyroid dysfunction. Thus, meticulous handling of hypothyroidism during pregnancy not only promotes fetal growth but also contributes to a smoother labor and delivery process.

Postpartum Thyroiditis and the Postpartum Period

Women with hypothyroidism face unique challenges during the postpartum period. Following childbirth, certain women may experience postpartum thyroiditis, which is marked by inflammation of the thyroid gland. Postpartum thyroiditis can initially lead to hyperthyroidism, as the body releases stored thyroid hormones into the bloodstream. After the hyperthyroid phase, the thyroid gland may become underactive, leading to hypothyroidism.

Postpartum thyroiditis may develop in women who previously had normal thyroid function prior to pregnancy, although it is more prevalent in individuals with a background of thyroid disease or autoimmune disorders. Postpartum thyroiditis symptoms may include fatigue, weight gain, depression, and a lack of energy. These symptoms can be difficult to distinguish from the typical exhaustion and emotional changes experienced during the early stages of motherhood.

During the postpartum period, women with pre-existing hypothyroidism may need to make adjustments to their thyroid hormone replacement therapy, it is important to closely monitor thyroid hormone levels and make any necessary dosage adjustments as the body goes through changes. Regular follow-up appointments with a healthcare provider are important for new mothers to maintain stable thyroid levels.

Breastfeeding and Hypothyroidism

Thyroid hormones play a crucial role in lactation. When dealing with hypothyroidism, it can occasionally disrupt milk production, causing challenges with breastfeeding. With proper treatment and monitoring, the majority of women with hypothyroidism can successfully breastfeed.

It is key to ensure that thyroid hormone levels remain within the normal range in order to support lactation. For women with hypothyroidism who want to breastfeed, it is important to follow the prescribed thyroid medication and discuss any concerns about milk supply with their healthcare provider. In certain situations, it might be helpful to seek guidance from a lactation consultant.

It's worth to mention that levothyroxine, which is the most

commonly prescribed thyroid hormone replacement, is considered safe to use while breastfeeding. The medication is present in breast milk in very small quantities, posing no risk to the baby. This enables mothers to maintain their treatment regimen while still being able to breastfeed.

Emotional and Psychological Factors

The emotional and psychological effects of hypothyroidism during pregnancy and the postpartum period can be quite substantial. Experiencing hormonal changes during pregnancy and childbirth, along with the physical demands of caring for a newborn, can intensify the symptoms of hypothyroidism. These symptoms may include fatigue, depression, and anxiety. These challenges can pose additional difficulties during the transition to motherhood and may impact the mother's ability to form a strong bond with her baby.

Postpartum depression is a significant condition that necessitates immediate treatment. It is crucial to assess the thyroid function of any new mother experiencing mood disturbances as part of the evaluation. Seeking counseling, joining support groups, and accessing mental health services can offer invaluable support during this period.

Healthcare providers should consider a comprehensive approach to care, taking into account both the physical aspects of hypothyroidism and the emotional well-being of the mother. It is important to provide new mothers with the necessary medical and emotional support to ensure their well-being and the well-being of their baby.

Long-Term Considerations for Mother and Child

With proper care during pregnancy and postpartum, women with hypothyroidism can expect a positive long-term outlook. Through effective management, the majority of women can experience successful pregnancies and give birth to healthy babies. Continued monitoring and care are critical to address any potential changes in thyroid function that may arise after giving birth.

During the early years of a child's life, brain development is of utmost importance, and maintaining proper levels of thyroid hormone is essential to facilitate this process. Infants born to mothers who effectively manage hypothyroidism during pregnancy generally do not encounter any thyroid-related complications. In situations where the mother's hypothyroidism was not properly managed or if the baby is diagnosed with congenital hypothyroidism, it is crucial to intervene and treat early to promote normal growth and development.

7.2. Co-existing Conditions

Living with hypothyroidism can pose challenges, especially when it coexists with other health conditions. Managing overall health becomes even more complex in such cases. The correlation between hypothyroidism and other diseases can have an impact on the intensity of symptoms, complicate treatment approaches, and influence one's overall well-being. Having a deep understanding of these co-existing conditions, especially autoimmune disorders and other prevalent health issues, is essential in order to develop a comprehensive approach to treatment and care.

Autoimmune Disorders and Hypothyroidism

Hypothyroidism often occurs alongside autoimmune disorders, particularly Hashimoto's thyroiditis, which is also an autoimmune condition. In autoimmune diseases, the immune system erroneously targets its own tissues, resulting in inflammation and harm. Managing hypothyroidism when it coexists with other autoimmune disorders can be quite complex. It requires careful monitoring and an integrated treatment approach.

Hashimoto's Thyroiditis: The Main Autoimmune Cause

Hashimoto's thyroiditis is a prevalent cause of hypothyroidism in the United States and numerous other countries. This condition results from the immune system targeting the thyroid gland, causing ongoing inflammation and ultimately impairing the gland's hormone production. Having Hashimoto's raises the chances of developing other autoimmune disorders, which is referred to as "autoimmune clustering."

It is not uncommon for patients with Hashimoto's thyroiditis to also have other autoimmune conditions, including rheumatoid arthritis, type 1 diabetes, lupus, or pernicious anemia. Diagnosing and treating these conditions can be quite complex due to the overlap of symptoms and the need to address multiple conditions at once.

Rheumatoid Arthritis

RA is an autoimmune disorder that primarily affects the joints, leading to pain, swelling, and eventually joint deformity. It is quite common for people with hypothyroidism, especially those with Hashimoto's thyroiditis, to also develop RA. There is likely a connection between the two conditions due to the immune system's tendency to target multiple organs and tissues.

Effectively addressing hypothyroidism alongside RA necessitates a well-coordinated strategy. Both conditions can result in fatigue, which can become worse when they occur together. In addition, certain medications used to treat RA, such as corticosteroids, may have an impact on thyroid function. It is critical to regularly monitor thyroid hormone levels in order to make necessary adjustments to thyroid hormone replacement therapy.

Type 1 Diabetes

Type 1 diabetes is often linked to hypothyroidism, another autoimmune condition. For type 1 diabetes, the immune system launches an assault on the cells in the pancreas responsible for producing insulin. This results in a shortage of insulin and elevated levels of blood sugar. People with type 1 diabetes have a higher likelihood of developing additional autoimmune conditions, such as Hashimoto's thyroiditis.

The relationship between hypothyroidism and type 1 diabetes can make blood sugar management more challenging. When metabolism is slowed down due to hypothyroidism, it may be necessary to make adjustments to the dosage of insulin. On the other hand, changes in blood sugar levels can impact thyroid function, leading to a complex cycle that needs to be managed with precision.

In order to effectively manage both conditions, it is crucial for patients to maintain close communication with their healthcare providers and regularly monitor their blood sugar and thyroid hormone levels. Integrated care, often involving experts in the field, is essential for maximizing treatment outcomes and minimizing the likelihood of complications.

Lupus

SLE is a long-term autoimmune condition that can impact different areas of the body, such as the skin, joints, kidneys, and heart. Similar to other autoimmune conditions, lupus is frequently found in individuals who have hypothyroidism, especially those who have Hashimoto's thyroiditis.

Diagnosing and managing lupus can be quite complex due to the overlapping symptoms it shares with hypothyroidism, such as fatigue, joint pain, and cognitive difficulties. In addition, lupus can lead to inflammation in the thyroid gland, which can further complicate thyroid function.

Successfully managing lupus and hypothyroidism necessitates a comprehensive and collaborative approach. Treatment typically includes immunosuppressive medications, which may interact with thyroid hormone replacement therapy. Consistent monitoring and open communication between healthcare providers are crucial for effective management of both conditions.

Pernicious Anemia

Pernicious anemia is a condition where the body struggles to absorb vitamin B12, resulting in a deficiency that can lead to fatigue, weakness, and neurological symptoms. It is commonly linked to hypothyroidism, especially in people with autoimmune thyroiditis.

Vitamin B12 plays a vital role in the production of red blood cells and the proper functioning of the nervous system. Insufficient levels can worsen the fatigue and cognitive issues that are already a part of hypothyroidism, making it more difficult to manage. Typically, treatment for pernicious anemia involves B12 injections or high-dose oral supplements, along with regular monitoring of thyroid function.

Additional Health Concerns Linked to Hypothyroidism

Aside from autoimmune disorders, hypothyroidism is frequently associated with other health conditions that can make its management more challenging. Having a deep understanding of these connections is crucial for delivering holistic care.

Cardiovascular Disease

There is a well-established connection between hypothyroidism and cardiovascular disease. Thyroid hormones have a significant impact on the regulation of heart rate, blood pressure, and cholesterol levels. When thyroid hormone levels are low, such as in hypothyroidism, there is an increased risk of developing heart disease.

People diagnosed with hypothyroidism tend to have elevated levels of low-density lipoprotein (LDL) cholesterol, commonly known as "bad" cholesterol. High levels of LDL can lead to the accumulation of plaques in the arteries, which raises the chances of developing atherosclerosis, heart attacks, and strokes.

Hypothyroidism can also contribute to bradycardia, a condition where the heart rate is slower than normal, and can worsen hypertension. Managing these cardiovascular risks necessitates a thorough approach, encompassing regular monitoring of cholesterol levels, blood pressure, and thyroid function. In certain situations, it may be necessary to include lipid-lowering medications or blood pressure treatments alongside thyroid hormone replacement therapy.

Depression and Mental Health Issues

Depression often accompanies hypothyroidism in many individuals. The connection between thyroid function and mood regulation is intricate, and insufficient levels of thyroid hormones can contribute to emotions of sadness, fatigue, and lack of motivation.

Depression symptoms can sometimes serve as an initial sign of hypothyroidism for certain individuals. After receiving a diagnosis, thyroid hormone replacement therapy can be beneficial in relieving depressive symptoms. However, it is important to note that certain individuals may still encounter mood disorders even after their thyroid levels have been regulated.

In these situations, it might be necessary to consider additional treatments, like psychotherapy. Healthcare providers should diligently observe patients for indications of depression and offer comprehensive care that encompasses their physical and mental well-being.

Obesity and Weight Management

Obesity is frequently linked to hypothyroidism. Having a sluggish metabolism due to low levels of thyroid hormone can pose challenges when it comes to shedding pounds, despite following a healthy diet and engaging in regular physical activity. Weight gain is a common symptom of hypothyroidism, and it can be quite challenging for many patients to manage.

Successful weight management in individuals with hypothyroidism necessitates a comprehensive approach. Although thyroid hormone replacement therapy can enhance metabolism, it may not be enough by itself to achieve substantial weight loss. A well-rounded approach that incorporates a healthy eating regimen, consistent exercise routine, and, in certain cases, the consideration of bariatric surgery might be required for certain individuals.

Addressing the psychological aspects of obesity is crucial, as weight gain can have a significant impact on self-esteem, mood, and mental well-being. Receiving assistance from healthcare providers, dietitians, and mental health professionals can greatly aid individuals in reaching and sustaining a healthy weight.

Gastrointestinal Disorders

The GI system can be affected by hypothyroidism, resulting in symptoms like constipation, acid reflux, and bloating. Metabolic processes slow down, which in turn affects the digestive system, resulting in a slower movement of food through the intestines.

Chronic constipation is a frequent issue for people with hypothyroidism, greatly affecting their quality of life. In certain situations, hypothyroidism may be linked to small intestinal bacterial overgrowth (SIBO) or celiac disease, which can potentially worsen gastrointestinal symptoms.

Addressing gastrointestinal symptoms in the context of hypothyroidism requires attention to both the underlying thyroid dysfunction and the specific gastrointestinal disorder. These may involve making adjustments to your diet, taking medications to enhance GI motility, and incorporating probiotics to promote gut health. It is important to regularly monitor thyroid function, as it can greatly improve GI symptoms by balancing thyroid hormone levels.

Sleep Apnea

Individuals with hypothyroidism are more prone to experiencing sleep apnea, a condition where breathing pauses during sleep. The relationship between the two conditions is intricate, as hypothyroidism may play a role in the development of sleep apnea due to factors like weight gain, muscle weakness, and diminished respiratory drive.

Sleep apnea can worsen the fatigue and cognitive difficulties linked to hypothyroidism, leading to a harmful cycle of inadequate sleep and deteriorating symptoms. Understanding and addressing sleep apnea is crucial for enhancing sleep quality and overall well-being.

Typically, sleep apnea treatment includes the utilization of continuous positive airway pressure (CPAP) therapy, which effectively maintains open airways throughout sleep. Weight management and thyroid hormone replacement therapy may be beneficial in mitigating the severity of sleep apnea symptoms.

Osteoporosis and Bone Health

If hypothyroidism is left untreated or not properly managed over a long period of time, it can lead to a decrease in bone density and raise the chances of developing osteoporosis. Thyroid hormones are involved in bone remodeling, which is the process of breaking down old bone and forming new bone. When thyroid hormone levels are low, this process can be disturbed, resulting in decreased bone strength.

Regular screening for osteoporosis is important for individuals with hypothyroidism, particularly postmenopausal women. Supplementing with vitamin D, in addition to engaging in weight-bearing exercises, is beneficial for preserving bone health.

Anemia

Anemia, including iron-deficiency anemia, is a condition that can occur alongside hypothyroidism. Chronic fatigue caused by hypothyroidism can be worsened by anemia, resulting in excessive tiredness, weakness, and impaired concentration.

Iron deficiency can disrupt the production of thyroid hormones, leading to a cycle where low iron levels worsen hypothyroidism and vice versa. Typically, treatment involves the combination of iron supplementation and thyroid hormone replacement therapy to effectively address both conditions at once.

Managing hypothyroidism can be challenging when there are other health conditions involved. However, by closely monitoring and taking a comprehensive approach to treatment, it is possible to effectively manage both the thyroid disorder and any associated health issues. Collaborating closely with healthcare providers to address every condition in a comprehensive manner is crucial for enhancing overall health and quality of life.

With a deep understanding of the connections between hypothyroidism and other conditions, individuals can proactively take steps to optimize their treatment, minimize the risk of complications, and improve their overall well-being.

8

Conclusion

As we come to the conclusion of this comprehensive guide on managing hypothyroidism, it's important to reflect on the journey we've undertaken through the pages of this book. Living with hypothyroidism is a complex, lifelong challenge, but as we've explored, it is a challenge that can be met with knowledge, careful management, and a holistic approach to health.

Throughout this book, we've delved into the intricacies of hypothyroidism, beginning with a clear understanding of what the condition is and how it affects the body. We've discussed how the thyroid, though small, plays a critical role in regulating metabolism, energy levels, and overall health. Understanding this foundational aspect of hypothyroidism is crucial because it sets the stage for everything that follows in the management of the condition.

We've also explored the various symptoms of hypothyroidism, both physical and cognitive. From the pervasive fatigue and weight gain to the more subtle but equally impactful symptoms like brain fog and mood swings, understanding the full spectrum of hypothyroid symptoms is essential for both patients and healthcare providers. Recognizing these symptoms early can lead to a quicker diagnosis and more effective treatment, preventing the long-term complications that can arise from untreated hypothyroidism.

Treatment, as we've discussed, is multifaceted. While thyroid hormone replacement therapy is the cornerstone of managing hypothyroidism, this book has emphasized that treatment goes beyond just medication. We've covered the importance of regular monitoring and adjustments to ensure that hormone levels remain within the optimal range. The role of diet and nutrition has also been highlighted, particularly how certain nutrients like iodine, selenium, and zinc are vital for thyroid function. Additionally, we've delved into the importance of physical exercise in boosting metabolism, improving mood, and enhancing overall well-being.

One of the key themes of this book has been the importance of a holistic approach to managing hypothyroidism. This means looking at the condition not just as a thyroid issue but as a health challenge that affects the entire body. We've discussed how lifestyle factors such as stress management, sleep hygiene, and environmental factors can all impact thyroid health. By addressing these areas, individuals with hypothyroidism can improve their quality of life significantly.

Special consideration has been given to the unique challenges presented by different life stages and co-existing conditions.

Whether it's managing hypothyroidism in children and adolescents, navigating the complexities of pregnancy and postpartum, or dealing with autoimmune disorders and other health issues that often accompany hypothyroidism, each stage and condition requires a tailored approach. The strategies provided in this book are designed to help individuals and their healthcare providers navigate these challenges with confidence and care.

As we close this book, it's important to offer words of encouragement. Living with hypothyroidism can feel overwhelming at times, but it's crucial to remember that with the right knowledge and tools, it is entirely possible to lead a full, active, and healthy life. The journey of managing hypothyroidism is not one that has to be taken alone. With a supportive healthcare team, a proactive approach to health, and the strategies outlined in this book, you can take control of your condition and improve your well-being.

In the end, managing hypothyroidism is about more than just addressing symptoms as they arise; it's about creating a lifestyle that supports your overall health and helps you thrive. By embracing a holistic, informed approach to your health, you can navigate the complexities of hypothyroidism and lead a life that is balanced, fulfilling, and vibrant.

Remember, your thyroid may play a small role in your body, but your approach to managing it can make a big difference in your life. Keep educating yourself, stay proactive in your care, and don't hesitate to seek support when needed. With determination and the right resources, you can live well with hypothyroidism.

Afterword

Glossary of Key Terms

1. Hypothyroidism: A condition in which the thyroid gland is underactive and does not produce enough thyroid hormones, leading to a slowed metabolism and various physical and mental symptoms.
2. Thyroid Gland: A small, butterfly-shaped gland located in the neck, responsible for producing hormones that regulate metabolism, energy levels, and overall bodily functions.
3. Thyroxine (T4): The primary hormone produced by the thyroid gland, which is converted into triiodothyronine (T3) in the body. It plays a crucial role in metabolism and energy regulation.
4. Triiodothyronine (T3): The active form of thyroid hormone, derived from the conversion of T4. T3 is more potent and is responsible for most of the biological effects of thyroid hormones.
5. Thyroid Stimulating Hormone (TSH): A hormone produced by the pituitary gland that regulates the production of thyroid hormones. Elevated TSH levels often indicate hypothyroidism.

6. Hashimoto's Thyroiditis: An autoimmune disorder and the most common cause of hypothyroidism, where the immune system attacks the thyroid gland, leading to its gradual destruction.

7. Thyroid Hormone Replacement Therapy (THRT): The standard treatment for hypothyroidism, typically involving synthetic thyroxine (levothyroxine) to replace deficient thyroid hormones.

8. Congenital Hypothyroidism: A form of hypothyroidism present at birth, which, if untreated, can lead to developmental delays and intellectual disabilities.

9. Subclinical Hypothyroidism: A mild form of hypothyroidism where TSH levels are elevated, but T4 levels remain within the normal range. It may or may not cause symptoms.

10. Levothyroxine: A synthetic form of thyroxine (T4) used to treat hypothyroidism by replacing deficient thyroid hormones.

11. Goiter: An abnormal enlargement of the thyroid gland, which can be caused by hypothyroidism, hyperthyroidism, or iodine deficiency.

12. Autoimmune Disorder: A condition in which the immune system mistakenly attacks the body's own tissues, as seen in diseases like Hashimoto's thyroiditis and rheumatoid arthritis.

13. Metabolism: The process by which the body converts food into energy. Thyroid hormones play a critical role in regulating metabolism.

14. Preeclampsia: A pregnancy complication characterized by high blood pressure and potential damage to other organs, often associated with poorly managed hypothyroidism.

15. Postpartum Thyroiditis: An inflammation of the thyroid gland that can occur after childbirth, leading to temporary hyperthyroidism followed by hypothyroidism.
16. Euthyroid: A state in which the thyroid gland is functioning normally, producing the appropriate levels of thyroid hormones.
17. Myxedema: A severe form of hypothyroidism characterized by swelling of the skin and tissues, often associated with untreated or poorly managed hypothyroidism.
18. Anemia: A condition in which the body lacks enough healthy red blood cells to carry adequate oxygen to tissues, sometimes associated with hypothyroidism.
19. BMR (Basal Metabolic Rate): The rate at which the body uses energy while at rest to maintain vital functions such as breathing and circulation, influenced by thyroid hormones.
20. Selenium: A trace mineral important for the conversion of T4 to T3 in the body, supporting thyroid function.

List of Sources

The information and insights provided throughout this book have been compiled from a variety of reputable sources, including peer-reviewed journals, clinical guidelines, and authoritative health organizations. Below is a comprehensive list of the primary sources referenced:

1. American Thyroid Association. "Hypothyroidism." Avail-

able at [thyroid.org](https://www.thyroid.org/hypothyro idism/).

2. National Institute of Diabetes and Digestive and Kidney Diseases. "Hypothyroidism (Underactive Thyroid)." Available at [niddk.nih.gov](https://www.niddk.nih.gov/h ealth-information/endocrine-diseases/hypothyroidism).

3. Mayo Clinic. "Hypothyroidism (Underactive Thyroid): Symptoms and Causes." Available at [mayoclinic.org](https://www.mayoclinic.org/diseases-condit ions/hypothyroidism/symptoms-causes/syc-20350284).

4. Endocrine Society. "Thyroid Disease." Available at [endocrine.org](https://www.endocrine.org/patient-engage ment/endocrine-library/thyroid-disease).

5. MedlinePlus. "Thyroid Diseases." Available at [medline plus.gov](https://medlineplus.gov/thyroiddiseases.html)
.

6. National Institute of Mental Health. "Depression: What is Depression?" Available at [nimh.nih.gov](https://www. nimh.nih.gov/health/topics/depression/index.shtml).

7. Thyroid Foundation of Canada. "Living with Hypothyroidism." Available at [thyroid.ca](https://www.thyroid.c a/living-with-hypothyroidism/).

8. Hormone Health Network. "Thyroid Disorders." Available at [hormone.org](https://www.hormone.org/disease s-and-conditions/thyroid).

9. Global Hypothyroidism Support Group. Available at [facebook.com/groups/hypothyroidism.support](https://www .facebook.com/groups/hypothyroidism.support).

10. PubMed and various peer-reviewed journals for scientific studies and clinical research articles on hypothyroidism and related conditions.